Living Your Passion

The 5 secrets to doing what you
love and LOVING what you do

By Keith Abraham

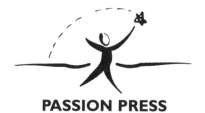

PASSION PRESS

Living Your Passion

The 5 secrets to doing what you love
and LOVING what you do
Keith Abraham

Passion Press
Keith Abraham
passion@livingyourpassion.com.au
www.livingyourpassion.com.au

To order the book, contact
passion@livingyourpassion.com.au

ISBN 0-9751993-0-7

Visit the Living Your Passion website at
www.livingyourpassion.com.au

What people think about Keith...

"I get to share the stage with a great variety of presenters... informative, inspirational, humorous and technical. But when Keith is on the programme I know it's going to be a stimulating session for he embodies all of the above. I admire people pursuing their dreams with passion. Keith's life is an extension of his passion and his presentations make both an impact and a difference. His value add and take away elements are uncomplicated and can be used immediately by the business groups he shares time with."

Max Walker, Sporting Legend, Author, Speaker

"In today's business environment we want more than just a speaker to inspire and inform us. We want them partner with us to provide us with innovative ideas and strategies to ensure that the presentation message lives on long after the conference has finished. Keith gives us unprecedented value and works with us to deliver a tailored solution for our organisation."

John Roca, Senior Manager, LEXUS AUSTRALIA

Keith alerted us to the need to change before we needed to and also stressed on the team importance of adopting an attitude which strives for constant improvement in everything we do. The workshop left us with a list of action items that we are currently progressing in order to take the business to the next level. Keith delivered a first class workshop and provided a great deal of material designed to help us strive for improved performance."

Ian Andrews, General Manager, Personalised Plates Queensland

What people think about Keith cont...

"I have had the opportunity to engage Keith Abraham on a number of occasions and in various organisations/industries I have worked. Keith is an exceptional presenter who has a great ability to acquire the knowledge of the business and to deliver a dynamic and engaging presentation to the audience. Keith stands out as a professional who delivers long lasting business results every time and from my perspective the return on investment through enhanced skill and personal development has been significant."

Mary Lindores, Human Resources Manager, IT Division, Woolworths Limited

"I LOVE getting your weekly motivator. I am sure, every week I receive it, I now DO it, instead of thinking about it. I have achieved more goals since I undertook your conference, then ever before."

Gayle Maria Warr, Conference Delegate, Telstra

"Keith was great value. He is a passionate and inspirational presenter. He gets through to people and really delivers. And what's more, he was a pleasure to work with, nothing being too much trouble. Keith's a real 'pro'."

Gary Evans, Manager - Human Resources, Credit Union Australia Limited

A passionate life is filled with moments, memories and pure magic.

Join the 3% Challenge...

You can't afford not to if, you want to live your life filled with success, wealth and achievement!

What you will receive...

- *Living Your Passion © Weekend Symposium*

Your 3 days of life-changing foundation growth with breakthrough experiences will lift you to a new level of success and achievement in your life and business. Be prepared...there will be no time to look back! In three days you will personally groomed in every area of your life. We assess YOU, Your Business, Your Career, Your Health and Your Wealth! This weekend is where you learn the 'mind skills' to make your wildest goals a REALITY.

(RRP $4950)

- *Living Your Passion © Definitive 12 CD Life Success Program*

1 year's Personal Success Programming, complemented by a 12 CD program + monthly activities. Keith will inspire you, motivate you and keep you on track for a full 12 months.

(RRP $2000)

- *3% Challenge © Executive Coaching Program*

Have your own personal coach 6 times a year to guide, challenge and keep you on track. Take control of your life and stay motivated and focussed with this 30 min tele-coaching sessions.

(RRP $1200)

- *The Ultimate 3% Challenge © Membership*

You will receive your own 3% Challenge Membership password to that will give you admittance to www.livingyourpassion.com.au website where you will have access to a panel of over 20 of Keith's personal success advisers to guide you towards your health, wealth and achievements - from Personal Trainers through to leading business authorities. You will also receive a monthly update newsletter with inspirational personal success stories and ideas on how to stay on track to achieve your ultimate life goals.

(RRP $2995)

Total Value = $10,555

Take The 3% Challenge Ultimate Package for only $5995.

No-Risk, No Questions Asked, No Hidden Catches, "Love it or your Money Back" Guarantee ... It's simple. Join us for our 12 month members of The 3% Club and if at any time during the program you're not 100% delighted with the value of the material, or you're not happy for any other reason just let us know and we'll give you a full refund. No hidden catches. No questions asked.

For more information email us, membership@keithabraham.com.au

Peak Personal and Professional Passion CD Series

Passion for Coaching CD Series

How to create loyal productive team members for your business

You will learn how to turn your team into a proactive and productive peak performance team. Using the 5 building blocks for guaranteed high performance, you will learn how to plan and conduct an effective sales team meeting. You will also understand the 5 ways to have a positive influence on your people and how to equip yourself to achieve outstanding coaching results. **RRP $319.** To order, visit our website www.livingyourpassion.com.au

Passion for Coaching Peak Performance Selling CD Series

You will discover

Why Leadership and Management are totally different; The Principles of Effective Sales Performance Coaching in Your Business; The 6 phases when developing an individual and the benefits of coaching; How to Plan and Conduct an Effective Sales Team Meeting with Your Team; The 5 Ways to Have a Positive Influence With Your People; Equipping Yourself to Achieve Great Coaching Results. **RRP $319.** To order visit our website www.livingyourpassion.com.au

Passion for Goal Setting CD Series

How to live your life filled with Power, Passion and Pizzazz

What you will discover - how to be passionate about your life and your business. You will learn the key elements of the goal setting process and how to set goals so you can stand out from the crowd. You will understand how to develop specific action plans to move you forward in the right direction and how to determine the things you value most in your life. You will define your long , medium and short term goals for your personal and professional life. You will also discover how to eliminate procrastination from your life by taking responsibility for your own happiness. **RRP $319.** To order, visit our website www.livingyourpassion.com.au

Passion for Conquering Change CD Series

8 insights on how to overcome challenges and conquer change in your life

What you will discover - how to equip yourself for changing times in order to evolve and move forward. You will learn the 8 steps to conquer your changing environment and to having a consistent, positive mind set. You will learn how to use change to your advantage by harnessing your potential to reach new levels. **RRP $319.** To order, visit our website www.livingyourpassion.com.au

Special Thanks

I would like to dedicate this book to my wife Kristine for her continual belief in me and her endless love and support. The memories we have created will last a lifetime but have also created our ideal life. Thank you.

To my two daughters, Mazana and Isabella, you fill my life with joyous adventures that I would not swap for anything. You are two of the most unique and special girls I know; may you always live your passion.

To Jill Price, my sister in-law who has been instrumental in the achievements we have had in our personal and professional lives. Thanks Jill, you are fantastic!

Every achievement I have accomplished has always been with the assistance of wonderful people, whether they be a family member, a friend, a mentor, a fellow author or a fellow speaker. I am so grateful that my life so far has been filled with these people who have inspired, challenged and motivated me to tap into my potential. Thank You!

Every journey is filled with challenges that build character. I am greatly appreciative to all of the people who have helped me through the challenges. Now, I can share and celebrate the successes with them.

Living Your Passion Foreword

Thank you for taking the time to read "Living Your Passion". You see, life is too short to live without a passion and too long to live with enduring mediocrity.

In the fast paced world that you live in, it is difficult to find the time to think about which vital steps should be taken to achieve all that you want out of life.

So I compliment you on spending the time and energy in investing in yourself, your dreams and your future.

I have a firm belief that you are your greatest asset. An asset that will not appreciate naturally with time, but will appreciate as you develop yourself, enhance your abilities, work on your attributes and live your passions.

My goal for you is simple. This book will be thought provoking, stimulating, inspiring and motivating. Most of all, I want this book to help you clarify your personal direction and to motivate you to take action towards discovering and living your passions.

Imagine if this book gave you one idea that made a positive difference in your life. This one idea creates a ripple effect in the lives of your family, your friends and the people you work with. The time that it takes to read a page, a chapter or the entire book will have been worth your time and energy.

I know that the principles in this book work. I have been the guinea pig for each and every principle I have outlined. I encourage you to not just read this book, but to complete and implement the exercises as you continue along your road of self discovery.

It is often said … "That life was not meant to be easy". My belief is life is meant to be an exciting journey. It is filled with life changing challenges and experiences, with the process leaving you with many memorable moments. Life is about LIVING YOUR PASSION.

Please enjoy. Sincere regards,

Keith

Keith Abraham

> "When you spend time, energy and money investing in yourself, you are a great judge of a sound investment."

Contents

Chapter 3 – Produce Your Plan

Chapter 4 – Progress Your Development

Introduction

Why this book ... Why now ... Why you?

Why were you created to achieve? I don't know you personally, but what I do know about you is that you where not born to go through the motions of life feeling unfulfilled, unsatisfied and unworthy. I don't know what happens to each of us during the journey called life, but we do lose our way.

Some of us find the pathway to personal fulfillment, happiness and success. For others, life becomes one task, one project and one job after another. It becomes boring, mundane, endless and empty. The question each of us needs to ask ourselves is ...

- ▸ "What is my purpose in life?"

- ▸ "What do I want to achieve?"

- ▸ "What do I want to do when I grow up?"

- ▸ "What is my passion and how do I pursue it?"

You may be reading this book for any number of different reasons. You may have drawn the line in the sands of life and said, "Enough is enough. I know what I don't want?" It could be that you have been an outstanding success and yet you are still not happy or satisfied. You may be asking yourself ... "What's wrong with me? I have everything I ever wanted, but I'm not happy." Maybe you just feel bored with your life and are wondering ... "Is this it for me?"

I don't know why you are reading this book, but no doubt you want an insight into yourself so that you can enhance your foresight and your future.

The most important question you can ask yourself is not only why you are reading this book, but what do you want to gain from this book? What insights do you want?

As you know, life gives us what we expect. Expect nothing, get nothing. Without an expectation, life gives us very little and we become disappointed when that happens.

> ### Designing Your Life by Robert Raftery
>
> **From today... let's dare to be different, let's direct that desire to change,**
>
> **To discover the height of real passion that a different direction can re-arrange,**
>
> **Designing your plan with a purpose, and with a real destination to pursue,**
>
> **Developing yourself on the journey, will connect with the genie in you.**
>
> **Now empowered with renewed determination, add discipline, then just do it!... Run rife!**
>
> **For when you stepped out and dared to be different,**
>
> **You started Designing your life!**

Are you designing your life?

One of the quotes that has had the greatest impact on my thinking over the past 15 years is ...

> # Most people spend most of their lives earning a living rather than designing a life.

How true is that for you? For me, it was very true. I lived from pay packet to pay packet, never thinking about what I wanted or where I was heading. You are rare if you haven't thought like this from time to time. Too often we earn a living without taking the time to stop and design the life we want to live.

I was 23 years of age when I first heard of the concept of goal setting. You see, I grew up on a farm and we didn't sit around the dinner table talking about goals, instead we talked about horses, cattle, trucks and tractors. At the time, I was going through the motions in a dead-end job. I knew I was not 100% happy, but I didn't know how to get out of the rut.

Before I had the opportunity to become a Professional Speaker and author, I had been employed in all types of positions, from my first job as a bricklaying labourer to senior management positions delegating to a staff of 65 people, 25,000 customers and responsible for a $15,000,000 budget.

When I dropped out of school the second time, I was employed in the prestigious position in the Local Council as a Noxious Weed Inspector! At this point of time you may be asking yourself, what does a Weed Inspector do? That is a good question! I was not very good at it nor was I dedicated to the position.

So here was an average day for me as a Noxious Weed Inspector. I would clock in at 8.00 am precisely. Then I would go to my desk and collect my official weed inspector clip board and the keys to my short wheel base, bright yellow Toyota 4WD. I would then inspect the Noxious Weeds growing along side the highway at over 100 kilometres an hour. That's no mean feat to any normal person!

At 9:00am, I would arrive at my morning tea destination, where I would have the recommended daily intake of vitamins, minerals and daily supplements for a Council Noxious Weed Inspector. This consisted of a can of coke, a vanilla slice and a cream bun.

Morning tea would conclude at 10 am sharp! I would then drive to remote locations where there were known noxious weeds and a lot of shady trees for a well earned two to three hour relaxation break of newspaper reading and sleeping.

I would awaken from my slumber and drive 30 minutes to my favourite lunch time destination - Goldstein's Pie shop! I would proceed to have a late lunch of Pie & Peas, after my fairly strenuous morning of about one and a half hours work.
I thought I was a pretty dedicated Council Employee. You see at

that time, I was keen to go above and beyond the call of duty for my employer using my special issue council binoculars to check that no official By-Laws were being broken at the beach by women bathing topless. Not that this was part of my role or this beach was even in my council area. I would then take a leisurely drive back to the office and clock out at 4 pm.

At this point of time you maybe asking yourself 3 questions ...

Weren't the weeds running rampant in my area? I don't know, it is difficult to tell when driving around at 100 km/h.

Secondly, what has a Noxious Weed Inspector got in common with you? Nothing! Except this one thing ...

If a pie eating, sleep all day, beach loving, high school drop out who was an unmotivated slob can tap into their potential, write a best selling book (Creating Loyal Profitable Customers – first published in 1999 and into it's 3rd reprint), become a recognised business development authority and a successful, in-demand, world travelled professional speaker, then imagine what you can do when you discover your passion and pursue it with purpose!

My story alone should give you hope! But hope without a plan is an empty promise.

The 3rd question which goes through people's minds is ... how do you go from a Pie Eating, sleep all day, Noxious Weed Inspector to International Conference Speaker and Best Selling Author? What happened to the Noxious Weed Inspector? Well let me tell you, it was a transformation, a transition and transmutation all rolled into one that has taken place over the past 20 years.

The first transition came when I was a 23 year old. My boss at the Albert Shire Council on the Gold Coast, came up to me one day and offered me the opportunity to attend a week long Leadership Program called RYLA – Rotary Youth Leadership Award. It was run by Rotary International.

Now as you can appreciate and understand, I was not a leader. I was in my comfort zone. I had dropped out of school and never finished year 12. My mum had got me my first job at the council. She had a lot of push in the Council as she was the tea lady! And now my boss wanted me to go on a leadership camp.

Then he mentioned the magic words … you get a week off work!

And I thought to myself, maybe I am leader! Maybe I'm a leader and I don't know it! Maybe I could be a leader for a week off work!

The week was fantastic. The defining moment for me was on the morning of the last day. The workshop presenter asked us to write 100 goals we wanted to achieve in our lifetime. I was 23 years of age and never heard about goal setting. The process seemed fairly simple at the time; you write out what you want and it comes true. He made us sit by ourselves for the next 60 minutes so that we could focus on writing down the 100 things we wanted to do in our lives. I diligently numbered the lines of my pages 1 to 100, ready to start.

Out of the blocks quickly, I wrote down 6 goals and then hit the wall. I was done. My mind was a blank. Dejected, I thought to myself that life is going to very short or very boring! It took a number of weeks, but I eventually wrote down 101 goals I wanted to achieve in my lifetime.

I didn't write down obvious goals. I wrote down things like ...

- Learn how to type.
- Learn how to swim
- Travel overseas and visit 100 countries.
- See a Cricket Test Match played in England.
- To be my own boss.
- To deliver a presentation to 1000 people.
- To be a professional speaker.
- Be happily married to a loving wife.
- Become a best selling author.
- Score a Hole-In-One at Golf.
- Own my dream car.
- Live on a golf course.
- Have beautiful children.

This one activity was the start of a positive chain reaction of events in my life that has shaped a life I could have only dreamt was possible. Has it been easy to do? No. Has there been challenges, setbacks and disappointments? Yes. But it is true to say that with any challenge there comes a greater appreciation for the achievement and rewards that are beyond your wildest dreams.

You see, your dreams can come true for you when you pursue them with a passion.

This book and the exercises I will suggest you do will take you to a new level of thinking; it will bring to the surface your true potential and turn that potential into reality.

You see, if it is not you that takes control of your life then who will? And if it is not now, then when?

If it is not you that is going to do it for you, then who is going to do it for you? Also, if now is not a good enough time to clarify your direction and your passion then when will it be a good time to do it? How much more pain and suffering do you have to go through before you say ... Enough is Enough!

Are you ready for your next adventure in your life? Start a new journey to discover your passion and live it.

CHAPTER I

PONDER YOUR PURPOSE

"If you don't stand for something,
you will fall for anything".

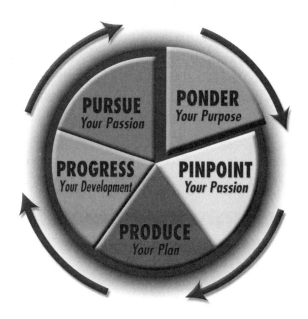

In this chapter you will discover ...

- How to define your lifetime purpose.
- Identify how to warm your heart, inspire your soul and revitalise your spirit.
- Answer the 7 questions to clarify your personal and professional purpose.

Your power comes from your purpose

Some men and women set out to change the world and others set out to be better parents to their children. Which is nobler? Neither. Both are equally important, it's just that one gains more publicity than the other. We often think of great deeds as those that are done by others on the global stage and are televised to us each night on the 6 o'clock news.

If the truth is to be told, it is far more important for you and I to fix our own backyards and to concentrate on fighting the battles we can win. It might be helping a child with their reading, so that they don't get teased at school. It could be taking the time to listen to a friend going through a challenging personal issue; it could be learning a new skill at an evening course; mentoring a work colleague on a business project or giving yourself the time to focus on what's important to you.

You have, believe it or not, so many purposes to choose from in your life. So never compare your purpose in life to that of others, unless you don't have a purpose at all. Most people do have a purpose but it is not defined.

I also believe that a purpose is developed with thought, it is clarified with experience and it is developed over time. You can have a number of different purposes at varying times of your life. You may achieve your purpose easily, you may never achieve it or you may change your direction from time to time and jump from one purpose to another.

Purpose comes in all shapes and sizes

Your purpose will come in all sizes of grandeur. As an individual you will have a purpose, but as a couple or as a family member you may have a different purpose. From my experience, you will most likely fit into one of these categories ...

- You may not have a purpose at all.

- You may have a purpose that is clearly defined that you are working towards right now.

- You may have once had a purpose but you achieved it and never considered the next purpose for yourself.

- You may have lost your purpose because you stopped focusing on it.

- You may have a professional purpose, but not a personal purpose. What I mean is, you know why you are in business or taking the career path you have taken, but personally what are you achieving with your family or with the people that count in your life? It may be the other way around i.e you have a personal purpose but no clearly defined purpose for your career or business.

- You may have fallen out of love with your purpose. In other words, you may love what you do but you are not in love with what you are doing at the moment.

What are you known for?
Your purpose, your passion or for your untapped potential?

Define your purpose

The solution to all of these situations is to simply take time out to clarify your purpose by completing the questions listed below. The definition of *Purpose* is to have a reason, a desire, an aim, an objective or intention. So let me ask you …

- What is your reason to get out of bed each day?

- What do you desire to be known for in your lifetime?

- What is one aim you want to achieve personally?

- What is one aim you want to achieve professionally?

- What is your current personal objective?

- Is it your intention to go through the motions of life or make something dynamic happen either for you, for your family, for your career, for your business or for your industry?

These are some of the questions you may want to ponder. Yes I appreciate that you need to earn a living, but what is the end goal for you, the big picture or the real reason to live? Your goals are just stepping stones towards your milestones on the pathway to your purpose.

People who do not have clarity of purpose find that their lives become mundane and boring. It becomes a task and a chore to complete every day. It becomes draining and they become exhausted, feeling like they are on a never-ending treadmill, without really knowing why.

Your purpose needs to warm your heart, inspire your soul and revitalise your spirit

If your answers don't warm your heart, inspire your soul and revitalise your spirit - then guess what? You're going through the motions if your answers are like...

- Pay the bills

- Just get by

- Because I have to

- I can't afford to retire yet

- I have customers to serve

- Put the kids through a good school

- I have nothing better to do with my time

What are your answers? Why do you do the things you do? The job you do? Stay in the relationships you stay in? Do you feel like you are going through the motions?

There was an old story that has always stayed with me. It is about 3 bricklayers constructing a wall. A passer-by asked them each the same question ... What are you doing? The first bricklayer replied, "What does it look like, I'm laying bricks!" The second said, "I am building a wall", and the third explained, "I am building a magnificent church that will stand the test of time and be used by thousand of families as a place of worship and celebration".

The stronger your purpose, the clearer the picture you have of your world.

So what could your answers have been?

- I am working towards becoming financially independent that will give me a great lifestyle of travel and time to pursue my other passions by the time I am 55 years of age.

- I want to lead an active life that contributes in a positive way to people I come in contact with each day. You could say I want to make a positive difference in people's lives.

- I want to be known by my customers as an exceptional customer service provider and recognised in my industry as someone to be benchmarked against.

- I want to provide a great educational experience for my children which lays a foundation for them to achieve whatever they want to do in their lives. For example: To fulfil their potential.

As an example; My current professional purpose is … To make a positive difference in the lives of people that I meet, to people that read my books and listen to my presentations and audio CD's. My personal purpose is … To be a great role model for my children, a loving partner to my wife, provide a great lifestyle for my family and be a positive person for my family and friends.

The companies and businesses globally that clarify their purpose are the ones that achieve, continue to grow and are recognised as market leaders. The businesses that fall from grace are the ones that forget about why they got into business in the first place or they became so internally focused that their vision is diminished to the point that they cannot see beyond their own self interests. The lesson we can learn from these examples is to take the time to create a picture of our purpose so that our subconscious can work on making it a reality.

The Next Step ...
Your Action Plan to Implement

- Take time to define your purpose for your life and list down in your personal journal or notebook.

- Complete the *Ponder Your Purpose Activity* on the following pages.

- Read your purpose statement every day for 7 days.

- After 7 days, alter or modify your purpose statement.

Action conquers inactivity

PONDER YOUR PURPOSE ACTIVITY

Writing a Purpose Statement is a process, it is not meant to
be mastered the first time you try. But, don't be surprised if you do.
The activity is simple and the questions will make you think.
The best way to tackle this activity is to write down your first
thoughts. Don't judge them or disqualify them - just write them
down. Once you have completed questions 1 to 6 then you will
be ready to complete question number 7.

1. How do you want to be remembered by your family?

_____

_____

_____

2. What is the one message, attitude or characteristic you want to
   leave with your children?

_____

_____

_____

3. What is the best way to teach that message, attitude or
   characteristic to your children without telling them?

_____

_____

_____

4. What have you become famous for in your work or in your business?

_____

_____

_____

5. What have you achieved in your career or industry?

_____

_____

_____

6. What don't you want to feel or be doing in your life, with
   your family, at your business or in your career?

_____

_____

_____

7. Take a moment now and write the first draft of your Personal
   and Professional Purpose Statement ...

_____

_____

_____

_____

_____

Personal Purpose Statement ...Professional Purpose Statement ...

_____

_____

_____

_____

_____

CHAPTER 2

PINPOINT YOUR PASSION

"How do you identify your true passion".

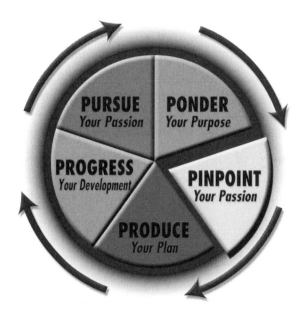

In this chapter you will discover ...

- How to do what you love to do in your life.
- Identify the characteristics every passionate person has and why you need them too.
- How to be in the top 3% of income earners in your country.
- The 8 ways to rekindle your passion for life.
- Answer the 9 thought provoking questions that will assist you in identifying your passions.

Passionate people are extraordinary!

Being a passionate person is not about being an Olympic Athlete or climbing Mount Everest. As individuals, I believe there are 3 levels in life that we operate on. The first is **Survival**, where you just get by but you don't get ahead. Have you been here? Do you know people like this?

The second is **Success**, where you are making progress but there is still the need to tap into your true potential. The third is **Significance**, where you are recognised by your peers and friends. You know in your heart that you are pursuing your passion and living a life worth living.

I believe the enemy of any personal progress is that our life is good, not great. Don't you deserve to be surrounding yourself with great successes and achievements as a result of tapping into your personal greatness?

We keep on doing what we have always done, for no other reason than it works. It's OK. It's good!

Too many of us suffer from **'sameness'**. We keep on doing what is comfortable, not what is going to give us a feeling of **completeness**. One of my strongest beliefs is that it is so easy to be extraordinary, because the majority of people lead ordinary lives.

Too many people put up with sameness. They go through the motions and are satisfied with the crumbs that life offers rather than taking the time to prepare for the banquets and feasts that can be enjoyed when you put yourself out of your comfort zone and dream big dreams, pursue your passions and set greatness as the standard to live by.

Passionate people love what they do!

Is it profitable to pursue your passion and love what you do?

I recall reading Robert J.Kriegel's book ... **If It Ain't Broke, Break It**. A number of years ago a study of 1,500 new workforce entrants starting their career were asked the above question with stunning results.

The researchers followed this group over a 20 year period. At the outset of the study, the group was divided into **Group A, 83% of the 1,500 people**, who were embarking on a career chosen for the prospects of making money in order to do what they wanted later. A path the majority of people, like you and I have been educated, instructed and informed to take in our own lives.

Group B, the remaining 17 percent of the sample, had chosen their career path for the exact opposite reason. They were going to pursue what they wanted to do now and worry about the money later. "How irresponsible", society, our parents and guidance councillors would tell us!

The data showed some startling revelations:

‣ At the end of the 20 years, 101 of the 1,500 had become millionaires.

‣ Of the millionaires, all but one - that is 100 out of 101 - was from Group B, the group that had chosen to pursue what they loved!

This research compliments that great quote from Mark Twain, the author of the all-time classic Huckleberry Finn, who said, "If you turn your vocation into your vacation, you will never work another day in your life".

Let me ask, **"Are you doing what you love to do?"** The question applies to both your personal life and your professional life. I am not asking you to leave your job; close your business down; leave your partner or spouse. I am not saying that your personal and professional life is going to be honky dory every single day.

But if it is not that way the majority of the time, then what are you doing to fix it? You need to address the roadblocks that are holding you back by taking control of issues and challenging your current circumstances.

It is often said that ulcers are caused not from what you have eaten, but by what's eating you. If you don't take time to pursue your passion, it eats away at you.

On the following pages there are 6 simple exercises to complete to assist you in identifying what you love to do. They will challenge your thinking. If you don't want to write in your book, then go to my website http://www.livingyourpassion.com.au Enter the Members only section and use the password: **takeaction** to download the different activities that are listed in this book.

Are you doing what you love to do?

ARE YOU DOING WHAT YOU LOVE TO DO ACTIVITY?

Please take a moment to ponder and then respond to the following questions. Follow your heart; write down your initial thoughts without pre-judgement or dismissiveness.

1. What would you love to do if you knew you could not fail? It's okay if you have more than one answer.

_____

_____

_____

2. What is one roadblock that is holding you back from achieving what you would love to do?

_____

_____

_____

3. How would you get around this roadblock if you had the time?

_____

_____

_____

4. What is one thing you need to do differently in your life?

_____

_____

_____

5. What is one small action step you could take in the next 24 hours that will make a difference in your life?

_____

_____

_____

6. What do you love to do that gives you back energy and recharges your batteries?

_____

_____

_____

> When people find their passion, they not only love what they do but they lead a life that other people only dream about.

The characteristics of passionate people ...

Are you one of them? My definition of a Passionate Person is someone who is following their heart towards their goals and dreams. They are doing what they love to do and are excited about their future. Passionate People are confident and content in the knowledge that they are in control of their own destiny. They are not perfect. Sometimes they feel out of balance, they still have challenging moments and they have doubts that sometimes cause them to stumble. But they get back up again to try and try again.

They are people just like you and me. They want happiness, to be loved, to have loved; they want acceptance and recognition from those who matter. I believe anyone and everyone can be passionate. Being passionate is not reserved for elite sports people or high profile achievers. It is part of those people's ethos and attitude that have a goal and to pursue it. It might be to pay off their mortgage in five years or to lose 5 kilos after their Christmas Holidays. Anyone can be passionate! It's a choice that you can make in a heart beat.

Following is a list of some of the qualities I have witnessed and seen in Passionate People as I have travelled around the world. **Give yourself a tick if you are or have been in the past one or more of these qualities and characteristics ...**

☐ I am Motivated

☐ I have a Positive Attitude

☐ I am Focused

☐ I have Healthy Self Esteem

☐ I have Personal and
Professional Goals

☐ I am Developing Myself
Personally and Professionally

☐ I Enjoy my Life

☐ I have a High Self Image

☐ I am Self Directed

☐ I Work to a Plan

- ☐ I don't Procrastinate
- ☐ I have High Energy Levels
- ☐ I am Enthusiastic
- ☐ I am Happy
- ☐ I am Solution Orientated
- ☐ I have Great Self Confidence
- ☐ I have a Love for Life
- ☐ I have Fun and Don't Take Myself Too Seriously
- ☐ I Laugh
- ☐ I Connect with People at all Levels
- ☐ I Listen and Absorb information
- ☐ I Love What I Do
- ☐ I Help People
- ☐ I set a Great Example for Others to Follow
- ☐ I Achieve and Get Things done
- ☐ I am Balanced and Level Headed
- ☐ I have Great Presence
- ☐ I make Eye Contact with People
- ☐ I am a Thinker
- ☐ I am Filled with Joy
- ☐ I stand up for my Values and Principles

It does not matter how many ticks you have. What it proves in my mind, as it should in yours, is that you are, you can be and you will always be passionate. What will vary is the level of feeling passionately about your life and your current endeavours. As you read this book, my goal is to give you the practical tools to maintain your level of passion to love your life and enjoy every part of it.

> The future is not some place we are going to, but one we are creating. The paths to it are not found, but made. And the activity of making them changes both the maker and the destination.

When did we lose the ability to dream?

Not so long ago my daughter, who was 5 years old at the time, told me that when she grew up that she was going to be a hair dresser, work in a clothes shop, be an actress and become a princess. Not in that order, by the way.

Her comments got me thinking. At what moment in time do we lose the ability to use our imagination? To go beyond the ordinary and dream big.

As children growing up we dreamed wonderful dreams, but as time goes by we can lose our ability to dream and to even become excited, enthused and energised about our achievements. It all seems too difficult.

The lives we live can be draining; they can feel like a series of personal bushfires we have to extinguish every day. But the question is; when are you going to stop, reassess and begin to do things differently? If you want things to be different then you must change the way you approach things in your life.

It is like the story of two men talking on the plane. One of the men asked the other, "How many times have you been married?" The other man replied, "10 times!" The other guy asked, "What was wrong with them all?"

My questions would have been, "What is wrong with you?" and "Who is the common element in 10 marriages?" You are the common element in everything that has ever happened to you in your life. Take responsibility and look inside.

IF I HAD MY LIFE TO LIVE OVER

I'd dare to make more mistakes next time. I'd relax, I would limber up. I would be sillier than I have been this trip. I would take fewer things seriously. I would take more chances.

I would climb more mountains and swim more rivers. I would eat more ice cream and less beans. I would perhaps have more actual troubles, but I'd have fewer imaginary ones.

You see, I'm one of those people who lives sensibly and sanely hour after hour, day after day.

Oh, I've had my moments, and if I had it to do over again, I'd have more of them. In fact, I'd try to have nothing else. Just moments, one after another, instead of living so many years ahead of each day.

I've been one of those people who never goes anywhere without a thermometer, a hot water bottle, a raincoat and a parachute. If I had to do it again, I would travel lighter than I have.

If I had my life to live over, I would start barefoot earlier in the spring and stay that way later in the fall. I would go to more dances. I would ride more merry-go-rounds. I would pick more daisies.

Nadine Stair

We can look outside ourselves but everything that affects you is about you. So if you want to change your circumstances, start to work on yourself. It is about moving from feeling helpless to becoming hopeful. I have always enjoyed reading the verse from Nadine Stair, an 85 year-old Kentucky women, who summarises what she would do differently in her life.

If it is too painful to address, then remember these simple philosophies during your lifetime...

- Life is too short and you are a long time dead!

- They can never pay you enough money if you hate your job.

- If you are doing this just for the children, remember they want you to be happy, not hampered in your life.

- Challenges can be temporary, unhappiness can be permanent.

Now on the other hand, it is fantastic if you are doing what you love to do. Make sure you pause from time to time to appreciate what you have. Remember the majority of people in society go through life without someone to love, someone to love them or a love for their life. Acknowledge and appreciate the job you do or the business you have. Be grateful and gracious with what you have achieved in your lifetime so far.

Now more than ever before, we need to be grateful for the successes we have achieved. We need to be our best friend, not our worst enemy. We need to nurture our spirit and soul because there are so many different elements that can wear us down every day.

LIVING YOUR PASSION SURVEY

Is passion one of the key ingredients you need to live a life that others will envy? You need to ask yourself the questions; "Do you have it? Are you pursuing your passion?" Take this quick survey to see if you are living your life to your full potential. Give yourself one point for every 'YES' you answer.

1. If someone woke you up in the middle of the night and asked you what your #1 goal was to achieve in the next 2 - 5 years, could you tell them in clearly defined terms?

2. Could you tell me one thing that you are most passionate about without having to think about it?

3. You make things happen and don't procrastinate?

4. Do you honestly feel you are working and making progress towards your long term goals?

5. Are you totally happy, satisfied and fulfilled in where you are going in your life?

Scoring System

If you scored the following points, then here is your prognosis.

0 = Do not despair - read on and find your true passion.

1 = No doubt about it, you have untapped potential ... it is now time to live your dreams

2 = Great ... you are right on track. Keep on pursuing your passion. Success and greatness is almost in your grasp.

3 = Fantastic ... Life is going to get better and better for you.

4 = Wow! You are making it happen ... Well Done!

5 = It is official ... you are a Passionate Person!!!

Are you passionate about your passions?

Very few adults ever set goals in their personal lives. Through my formal and informal research from working with over 165 companies and speaking to over 100 conference groups each year for the past 8 years, I can testify to this fact.

Sure people have business goals and targets to achieve, but most of the time these objectives are given to them by their management team or Board of Directors. Every high achiever or individual I have met or worked with in my capacity as a hired leading authority has had a goal.

It is no secret that people who set their goals achieve more, regardless of the type or scale of goals they pursue. I won't say that they are more balanced or live longer, but they are more fulfilled, happier for longer periods of time and much more satisfied with their lot in life. This one observation makes them different from the majority of people that you and I know.

It is often said that for every 100 randomly chosen people, each would most likely fit into one of these 4 areas ...

3% of these have firm written goals with action plans to achieve them. These are the people who make things happen.

10% of these people have firm goals that are not written down. These people think or expect things to happen.

60% of these people have vague or limited goals. They spend more time planning to go on their next holiday. These people are the ones who watch things happen.

27% of these people go through life with no goals at all. These are the people who don't know what happened!!! They ask "Where did my life go?"

There have been a number of studies done where they have tracked people for over 20 years after the initial survey was done. It was interesting to note that the majority of people in the 27% category were on some type of welfare payment. The group belonging to the 60% were earning the average weekly wage from a job. The people in the 10% of all of the people surveyed were earning 3 times the average weekly wage and the top 3% of people were earning 10 times the average weekly wage.

Now what do you think; is goal setting worth it?

It is always your choice which category you fit into. All you need to do is decide what your goals are, define them and start doing something about it. It is easy to be different, just do what other people don't do, refuse to do or ignore. This will make you different in a positive, productive and proactive way.

Life is too short to live without passion and too long to live with mediocrity.

Putting your passion into practise

Some time ago now I was speaking at a conference in North Queensland at the Capricorn Resort. This resort has 2 magnificent golf courses. As I was waiting in the hotel lobby for my transfer back to the airport, I met a really interesting guy in his early 50's. Firstly, he looked interesting, dressed in his Plus Fours golf pants, colourful shirt and golf shoes. We got chatting and he asked me what I did, and I replied that I was a professional conference speaker who talked about helping people to live their passion. He replied, "I know what you mean."

As we talked further he explained that at long last he was starting to live his passion. I asked him about what he did. He explained that he was once a senior manager with a global insurance company, travelling all over the world, managing thousands of people, in charge of millions of dollars and felt totally miserable. The turning point came when he woke up one morning in a hotel room but couldn't remember what city he was in. His life had become a blur. Upon his return, he told his wife of 25 years that things had to change. She told him that she still loved him, but he was unhappy, miserable to be around and that he was no fun at all.

She asked him some simple but thought provoking questions ... "What would you love to do for a job or a business?" He jokingly replied to his wife, "Well I love golf and eating fine food!" Now knowing that he was not a professional golfer, he was not on holidays at the resort and had not yet retired, I started to become inquisitive about his journey from miserable senior manager to being at Capricorn Resort playing golf. So I asked the question again,

"What do you do now?" He replied that he had combined his 2 passions in life, eating fine food and playing golf to create a business that organised Gourmet Golf Tours for people. They travelled all over the country wining, dining and playing golf. He mentioned it didn't pay as much as his last job but he was a thousand times happier.

This example demonstrated to me that by using your imagination you can design a life and earn a living around your passion. The benefits being that you will be eternally happy and internally wealthy.

> When people find their passion, they not only love what they do but they lead a life that other people only dream about.

What are you passionate about in your life?

The answer always lies in the quality of the questions you ask yourself. People often tell me that they don't know what their passion is or what goals they want to achieve and that's OK. Few of us ever take the time to think about our future. We don't ponder the questions that will equip us to grasp our futures.

Here are the questions that will start you thinking about what your passions are. Then you can identify how to pursue them in the following chapters in this book.

- What does having a Passion mean to you?

- What was one thing either in the past or present that you were passionate about, really focused on or just loved to do?

- If you won 10 Million Dollars in Lotto tomorrow, what would you love to do with your time and energy?

- Of all the things you have ever done, what were you doing when you were the happiest?

- What are the five things that you value the most in your life?

- In 30 seconds, write down the three most important goals in your life right now.

- What have you always wanted to do but been afraid to attempt?

- What type of activities or circumstances give you the greatest feeling of importance?

- What is the one thing which you would dare to dream if you knew you could not fail?

With passion comes the energy to excel

Life is too short to get up, go to work, come home, have an alcohol injection and go to bed cranky. Especially if you repeat the same pattern on a daily basis.

Let's take the focus off your business or career, because they can be so difficult to change sometimes. Have you ever noticed that when you are doing things you love to do, that time seems to evaporate before your very eyes?

But on the upside, you always seem more energised for undertaking that activity. When you do the things you love to do, you recharge your batteries, re-energise your enthusiasm and rekindle your spirit.

Yes, it is true that you will never get back that time but what you will receive in return is the energy to plough on, face challenges and overcome obstacles. You will have the one critical ingredient to be a better partner, spouse, father, mother, son, daughter, friend, business person, employee or manager ... **ENERGY!**

Look at it this way. Each of us have a rechargeable battery in our body and from time to time it goes flat. How do you recharge it? What do you do to recharge your batteries? The simple answer is to take time to do the things that you love to do. It may be fishing, going to the movies, having a few drinks with your friends, watching the football, having an afternoon snooze, enjoying coffee and cake at you local café, reading a novel or watching your favourite movie.

You cannot give what you do not have!

From time to time we all need to escape and reconnect with ourselves. There are things you can do in moments and minutes and there are activities that will take hours or even days. The question is; what will do it for you and when are your going to do it next? Remember our conscious and sub-conscious perform positively when they have something to look forward to in the future.

On the downside, if you don't stop from time to time to recharge your batteries, you become lethargic and unmotivated. At the same time, your body, mind and spirit become so run down that you become susceptible to fatigue and life threatening diseases.

If you are having difficulty with taking big chunks of time off, then every day give yourself just 1% of that day - just 15 minutes. I know you can find 15 minutes for yourself. There are lots of things you can conquer in 15 minutes ... go for a quick walk to wake up the mind and body, do your own circuit workout in the garage at home or read a positive, uplifting book. Did you know that if you read for 15 minutes a day you would read 8 to 10 books a year? What about 15 minutes of meditation, yoga or Pilates? Take 15 minutes to reconnect with your children by reading a story, helping with a project or talking to them about their day.

How to rekindle the passion within?

You may be a passionate person, but at the moment you are dispassionate. From time to time, you will lose passion for the goals you want to achieve or the direction you have taken. It happens to all of us.

In my business, I love what I do, being a writer and speaker at conferences. But about 12 months ago, I felt dispassionate about my business and my career. I loved what I did but I was not in love with what I was doing. A mentor, Dr. Keith Maitland asked me these questions ... "What's your purpose in life? Why do you do the things you do?" I went away and answered his questions which were the catalyst for getting me focused again.

So I thought I would provide you with some thoughts that will rekindle the passion within so that you can achieve your goals.

- Clarify your purpose and rewrite your goals
- Write down 100 things you want to do in your lifetime
- Take a holiday and recharge you batteries
- Talk about your feelings with a friend or mentor
- Find a short term objective to focus on
- Obtain a feeling of achievement
- Go and do some activities you love to do
- Find a new challenge to break the boredom

Everyone can be passionate; it's just sometimes your passion needs to be rekindled.

The power of your passion will pull you towards your destiny.

The Next Step ...
Your Action Plan to Implement

- Take time to answer the 'Doing what you love' survey.

- List down 3 dreams in the past that you have given up on achieving.

- Complete the 9 'What are you passionate about?' questions.

- Identify one action you are going to take in the next 7 days to rekindle your passion and the ability to dream.

Don't be intimidated by your ideas, initiate your ideas.

CHAPTER 3

PRODUCE YOUR PLAN

"How to bring your passion into reality"

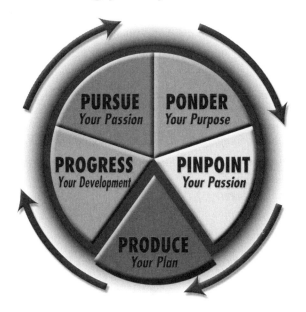

In this chapter you will discover ...

- The 4 key stages of the goal setting process.
- Identify how to turn your passions into long and short term goals.
- Understand what true personal success means to you.
- The 8 key areas to set your goals in your life.
- Ten ways to remain focused on the things that count for you.

Goal setting is simple, when you know where to start

Everyone talks about how you should have a goal. You must set goals. Few people if anyone, give you the step by step processes to collect your thoughts and then turn them into a tangible action plan that is directed towards your purpose. Try to find a book on the "How to's" of goal setting and you will struggle. One of reasons I was compelled to write this book as practically as possible is to give you the knowledge and the tools to turn your purpose and passion into realistic goals.

There are 4 stages to the goal setting process as the following model describes ...

The 4 Goal Setting Stages

1. CREATION	2. SPECIFICATION
3. IMPLEMENTATION	4. CELEBRATION

The first stage is *Creation*; this is where you create your long, medium and short term goals. It is your opportunity to dream about what is possible; it is about letting your mind run wild and digging into your heart to release your internal desires. Dreams are what goals are made of in your life.

The second stage is **Specification**; it is about taking the time to specify exactly what you want to achieve. The power of any goal is in how vividly you can create it in specific terms. In this section, you will clarify your goals and the time frame in which you wish to achieve them.

Implementation is the third stage. This is where the rubber meets the road. Nothing ever happens until someone implements the plan. Goal setting is easy. It is remaining focused on your goals that is the hard part. I will share with you some easy to implement techniques to make sure your goals come true.

Finally, the fourth part is **Celebration**. It is critical to celebrate your successes. If you are going to work your brains out to obtain your goals, then don't you deserve to celebrate? It is important for your sub-conscious to feel the benefit of success.

> Your life can either be a daring pursuit of your goals or a hollow excuse of what could have been.

Creating your long term goals

There have been many great stories told about Walt Disney and the adversity he overcame to create Disneyland, the movie company and the business empire that extends all around the globe. But my favourite story happened after he passed away on the 15th December, 1966. It was the opening day of Walt Disney World in Orlando, Florida on the 1st October, 1971 and Roy Disney, Walt's older brother, was walking all the media through the park prior to the arrival of the guests, explaining why Walt wanted the Magic Castle here and why this particular attraction was placed there.

It was then that one of the journalists made the offhand comment to Roy Disney, "Isn't it a shame Walt never got to see this place open?" Roy stopped in his tracks and looked the journalist in the eye and said, "The reason why you and I see it today is because Walt saw it first". It is no wonder that one of Walt Disney's favourite quotes was ...'If you can dream it, you can do it'. His imagination created the vision and he then turned his vision into a reality. That is the essence of goal setting!

What goals do you have for your future? What visions do you want to turn into a reality? What could you achieve if you knew you would be triumphant in your quest to achieve that goal?

If you never know your passion, you will never fulfil your true potential.

What don't you want in your life?

I often ask the question to people in presentations, workshops and in general conversation, "What do you want to achieve?" Only to have the reply given back to me, "I don't know!" Which then prompts to ask the annoying question, "Yes, but if you did know what would you like to achieve?" When that fails, as it often does, I ask the fool proof question, "What don't you want?"

It never ceases to amaze me that people can tell what they don't want, but can't tell me what they do want. Participants in my day long, **Living Your Passion Workshop** will often tell me in private that they hate their jobs. This leads me to ask them what type of job would they love to do and when the response is, "I don't know!", my response is simple - "You deserve the job you have!"

If you don't know, then that is OK! However, to not have thought about what the alternatives are is not acceptable. It is sometimes easier when you don't know what you want and then reverse that situation to discover what you do want. If you don't want a boring job working with these types of customers, then ask yourself what would be an exciting job? What aspects would a job have that would make it exciting to you? Does it involve travel, meeting different types of people all the time or new challenges on a regular basis?

Think about the alternatives to your current situations. Stimulate your mind, look at your options and challenge your thinking.

100 things you want to do in your lifetime

As I mentioned in an earlier chapter, one of the defining moments in my life was when I was asked to list down 100 things I wanted to achieve in my lifetime. My initial thought was it was going to be too easy, but as I undertook the challenge I was surprised at how little I wanted to achieve or how few things I could think of to do in my lifetime.

It was only 6 things initially and at that point I thought my life was going to be very short or very boring! However after a couple of attempts, I finally got 101 things written down and since then I have done this exercise three times. This one activity, as simple as it seems, is liberating, challenging and energising.

Not long after attempting this exercise I read a story in LIFE Magazine about John Goddard. He was deemed ... 'The Great American Dreamer'. As a boy of 15, he overheard his Uncle and Father talking about their lives and noticed a sense of unfulfillment in his Uncle's voice. It was at that moment he put down his homework and wrote out a 'Life To Do' list ... 127 goals that he wished to accomplish in his lifetime. He wanted to explore The Nile and Amazon Rivers, climb Mt. Everest, learn to fly a plane, dive in a submarine, learn how play the flute, type 50 words a minute, have an article published in National Geographic, compose music, read the complete works of Shakespeare, Plato, and Aristotle, visit a movie studio, just to mention a few. He is now 74 years of age and has accomplished 109 of his 127 goals.

It is a wonderful activity for exercising your imagination and starting to channel your thinking. It is not about being right, it's about dreaming, thinking and inspiring you to believe that whatever you imagine, you can achieve. It is about planting seeds in your subconscious so it can recognise the opportunities that will produce the right scenarios for you to generate positive outcomes.

So here is your challenge. Obtain a journal or lined book and ask yourself these questions to create your list of 100 Things you want to do in your lifetime.

- What do I want to do in my lifetime?
- What type of person do I want to become?
- What do I want to see in my travels?
- What would I like to contribute to others?
- What do I want to achieve in my lifetime?
- What adventures have I completed?
- What financial goals have I conquered?

If you find this exercise tough going, that is OK. It is not until you tap into your inner thoughts that you will be surprised and inspired by your writing. It may take you a couple of sittings to get your list of 100 or perhaps you may nail it in your first attempt.

Having a passion is more about your ability to dream of what could be, rather than dwelling on what could have been.

Here are some more examples that may assist you in starting your list ...

› Scuba Diving	› Write a Book
› Go Whale Watching	› Take the Orient Express
› Learn how to Ski	› Learn how to Cook
› Visit Disneyland	› Ride a Harley
› Go on an African Safari	› Swim with Dolphins
› Play Golf at Augusta, USA	› Become Debt Free
› Be in a Stage Play	› Paint a Picture
› Fish for Blue Marlin	› Own Your Dream Home
› Visit the Pyramids	› Live until You are 100+

These are some of the areas you may want to think about when your start dreaming about your Passions and Goals for the future ...

› Career	› Contributions to Society	› Adventure
› Recreation	› Knowledge	› Toys
› Relationships	› Social Activities	› Family
› Education	› Travel	› Home
› Financial	› Business	› Holidays
› Personal Growth	› Health	› Lifestyle
› Community Service	› Sport	› Hobbies
› Investments	› Fitness	› Friends
› Motor Cars	› Spiritual	› Boats

> # Life is just not about pursuing your passion one day; it's about having a passion every day.

Your definition of true personal success

Some time ago I created a formula for setting goals that looks like this ...

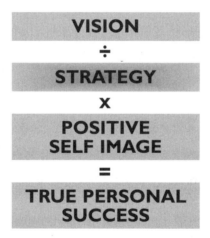

VISION

÷

STRATEGY

x

POSITIVE SELF IMAGE

=

TRUE PERSONAL SUCCESS

Your **Vision** divided by your **Strategy** and then multiplied by your **Positive Self Image** equals **True Personal Success**. You see, if you have a Vision but no plan, you have only a wish. The great multiplying factor of this equation is your level of Self Image. You cannot out-dream your esteem. If you don't believe you can achieve that goal, then you won't. If you don't believe you are worthy, then you aren't.

However, in making this formula work for you, it is critical to start with the end in sight. What is your definition of True Personal Success? Is it happiness? Is it freedom to do as you please with your time? Is it helping others? Is it becoming financially independent? Take a moment now and define what success means to you. It can be a word, a statement, a sentence or even lists of ideas.

What types of goals should I have?

I am repeatedly asked this question. There are a number of different areas in which you can set goals to live your passion. The 8 areas I recommend that you can focus on when setting your goals initially are these ...

1. **Career/Business**

2. **Financial**

3. **Family**

4. **Community**

5. **Health & Fitness**

6. **Personal Growth**

7. **Adventure**

8. **Lifestyle**

Career / Business Goals

Relate to the goals you want to achieve during your working life whether as an employee or in your own business. It is the positions or roles that you have want to obtain or the achievements you want to be recognised for in your business.

Financial Goals

These goals are to do with either the income you want to earn, the money you want to save or the investments you want to acquire. Think about what financial situations you want to change or have or the results you want to obtain.

> There are many things in life that catch your eye, but only a few things will catch your heart... pursue those with a passion.

Family Goals

I am great believer in having goals as a family. Whether they are activities that you want to do together or characteristics that you want to have as a family. Families take energy and effort to make them work well. This is one area that deserves a superior investment of time.

Community Goals

You and I can contribute to our friends and to our community in a number of different ways. You must decide whether it is through the giving of our time or money. Maybe your contribution to the community is looking after the under 9's soccer team, organising your 20 year school reunion or welcoming a new neighbor to your street with a cup of coffee. What do you want to contribute?

Health and Fitness Goals

This is one area that everything else revolves around. It's hard to achieve great things when you are sick. These goals relate to you energising your body, mind and spirit, so that you can feel great.

Personal Growth

As you enhance your self esteem, you also enhance your ability to believe in yourself and what you can achieve. What additional skills and knowledge do you want to obtain? What attitudes do you need to reprogram in your mind? These goals could involve you going back to school or be as simple as reading a book that will enhance your self esteem and self confidence.

Adventure Goals

Adventure could be about going parachuting or it could be about sitting on a white sandy beach sipping huge cocktails whilst having a relaxing island holiday. These goals are the places you want to visit, the things you want to see and the activities you want to do.

Lifestyle Goals

It is not necessarily about imitating lifestyles of the rich and famous, but it can be. This area involves two parts ... the first is what you give to yourself and family in the way of gifts and rewards. The second is what you give back to yourself. I mentioned in a previous chapter that everyone has a 'battery' that we need to recharge from time to time. Lifestyle goals give you back the energy to keep on doing what you want to do with vigor and vitality, whether it's taking time out to play sport or to pursue a hobby.

> To pursue your passion and never achieve it is far better than never having a passion and living with regret forever.

Long Term – Medium Term – Short Term Goals

I classify long term goals as 10 year goals and medium term goals as goals that are 5 years from now. Your short term goals are goals that you would like to achieve in the next 12 months. I encourage you to complete the next two exercises in your journal or exercise book. First divide your page into 8 parts. These areas represent the 8 areas you want to set your goals in. It does not matter if you do not have goals in all 8 areas of your life for the next 10 years or even 5 years for that matter. This is one activity that is designed to help you clarify what is important for you to focus on in the next 5 to 10 years. It is also an opportunity to review your list of 100 things you wish to achieve in your lifetime, so you can determine where they fit in your master plan.

Long and medium term goal setting questions

Now if your think 10 years is too far away, then think about your age and then add 10 years. Scary, isn't it! Now do you think the last 12 months have gone pretty quickly? Yes? Then I rest my case. Your life will pass you by before you know it. Answer these questions in your journal or exercise book.

‣ **Where do I see myself in the next 10 years?**

‣ **What do I want to be doing in the next 10 years?**

‣ **What do I want to have achieved in the next 10 years?**

‣ **What type of person should I become in the next 10 years?**

‣ **Where do I want to go in my travels in the next 10 years?**

‣ **What is my financial position in the next 10 years?**

Now repeat the exercise for the next 5 years in your journal or exercise book.

‣ **Where do I see myself in the next 5 years?**

‣ **What do I want to be doing in the next 5 years?**

› What do I want to have achieved in the next 5 years?

› What type of person will I become in the next 5 years?

› Where do I want to go in my travels in the next 5 years?

› What is my financial position in the next 5 years?

Some people dream and never do. Some people are always doing and never dream. Some people do both and are living their passion!

What do you want to achieve in the next 12 months?

Some people find it easy to write down their 10 year goals and difficult to write down their 5 year goals. Others find it harder to think about what they want to be doing in 10 years. Whatever your experience, it is now time to think about your short term goals for the next 12 months. Once again, use your journal or exercise book to answer the following questions in each of the 8 goal setting areas.

Career / Business goals for the next 12 months ...

- What would you like to achieve in your career?
- What type of roles do you want to be doing in your career?
- What would be a great job to do or business to own?
- What would you like to achieve in your business life?

Financial goals for the next 12 months ...

- How much money do you want to earn in the next 12 months?
- How much do you want to save or invest?
- Which debts do you want to retire in the next 12 months?
- What personal financial circumstances do you want to change?

Community goals for the next 12 months ...

- What would you like to contribute to your community?
- What would like to do for your friends in the next 12 months?
- What activities would you like to be involved in for your community?

Family goals for the next 12 months ...

‣ What would you like to achieve as a family in the next 12 months?

‣ What would you like to do for your family?

‣ What type of person are you going to become for your family?

Health and Fitness goals for the next 12 months ...

‣ How fit and healthy would you like to be in the next 12 months?

‣ What is your fitness goal for this year?

‣ What are some of the fitness activities you would like to pursue?

Personal Growth goals for the next 12 months ...

‣ What activities are you going to do in the next 12 months to develop your skills, knowledge and attitude?

‣ What courses are you going to do to improve yourself?

‣ What do you want to do to become a better person?

Adventure goals for the next 12 months ...

‣ What type of holiday would you like to take?

‣ What type of adventure activity would you like to do?

‣ Which one of your goals from your list of 100 things are you going to complete in the next 12 months?

Lifestyle goals for the next 12 months ...

‣ What are you going to do just for you?

‣ What rewards are you going to give you or your family?

‣ What revitalises you, gives back energy and recharges your batteries?

Easy Road or the Hard Road. Which road will you take?

Goal setting is easy to do if you know how and are prepared to take the hard road. What's the hard road? It is doing what most people refuse to do. By taking this path, you can have what the majority of people will never experience in their lifetime; success, achievement, fulfillment and true happiness.

It is about doing the tough things, taking on the challenges and having a go; it is about taking time out to set your goals. The easy road is to put it off. The majority of people say, "I know all about goal setting, I will write out my goals on the weekend or when I get a spare half an hour."

That time never arrives and the activity never happens because we are all too busy being busy. The hard road is about physically sitting down, turning off the TV, closing out the interruptions and asking yourself the questions on the previous pages. It is easy to take the easy road and to procrastinate.

I don't think we should be selfish, but I do believe we need to put ourselves at the top of the list sometimes. Get yourself right and your life will become simpler. If you don't address the obvious challenges, then how can you possibly feel true happiness or a love for life and reach your 'well' of untapped potential?

Rechelle Hawkes, the captain of the Women's Olympic Hockey Team, was asked why they put so much effort into winning a Gold Medal when there are no guarantees that they will be selected for the game or even win the tournament.

Her reply was simple …

"We Choose To Do This Not Because It Is Easy, But Because It Is Hard." Rechelle Hawkes – Captain Australian Women's Hockey Team, Double Gold Medalist, Triple Olympian

The point I took from her reply was that if it is worth doing, it will be hard, otherwise we would all be Olympians. We would all win gold medals.

To experience triumphant you must first pursue your passion.

Target In On Your Goals

Now that you have created your dream list, it is time to set about making them come true for you. Too many people have a dream but they never take the time to clarify what it is that they really want from life. Always dreaming, never getting around to the doing. They are always striving, but they never arrive and this means they are never able to thrive. The simple formula I use can be easily remembered by thinking about your goals as targets.

TARGET stands for …

Target Defined

Action Plan Developed

Realistic Time Frame

Get Focused

Enjoy the Journey

Take Time to Dream, Again

Target Defined

Remember vague goals equal vague results, so it is critical to specify exactly what is it you want to achieve. During my one day workshops, participants will often say to me, "I want to make more money this year than I did last year!" My reply is "OK, I will personally speak to your boss and have them increase your income package by $1.00 per annum. Your goal will be achieved!" For some unusual reason, people don't see the funny side of that gesture. But you have to be so careful, clear and concise with what you want to achieve because the universe will provide you with what you expect. If your expectations are low or vague then your results will be minimal, achievements low and your successes small.

Once you have written out your goals, go back and review each one of them to check if they are clearly defined. The true test is to ask yourself if a magic genie came along to grant your wishes, could they understand exactly what you meant when they read your goals, or would they be unsure about what you really wanted to achieve.

You see our subconscious operates best when it is given clarity. A target ensures it won't be confused and that we don't become inactive. You will be unshackling one of your greatest assets and its ability to dream, imagine, believe and identify the many opportunities that can make your dreams come true. To give you a better understanding of this concept, look at these examples and see what you think this person really wants to achieve ...

- I want to get a new job.
- I want to start an investment account this year.
- I want to save more money this year.
- I want to improve my personal relationships with my partner.
- I want to lose some weight and get fit.
- I want to have a good holiday this year.

I know all of these goals are vague and, if you are honest with yourself, you have at some point wished or dreamt about achieving goals like this without really clarifying exactly what it is you want. I know I have done it. Take the time to be specific. The moments that it will take you to clarify and specify will save you days, weeks, months and even years of frustration. When things don't happen fast enough for you read over your goals.

Here is an amended example … **I want to get a new job.**

> ‣ I want to be in a new role as a Business Development Manager in the mortgage industry earning $60,000+ by the 31st May, 2005. The company that employs me will be one of the major players in the market place. (You could even be specific which company it is.) They will provide me with a company car, the freedom to be creative and innovative in a dynamic fun team environment with opportunities to progress further in my career. (Be even more specific by listing down the location where you want to work.)

To assist you to create greater clarity in your goals, here are some questions you can use as a clarifying mechanism. These are quality questions you need to ask yourself to not only clarify your goals but to confirm and convince yourself that this is the goal for you …

> ‣ How much money do you want?
> ‣ How much money will you need?
> ‣ How much time will it take?
> ‣ How long before you want it to happen?
> ‣ What type of role do you want to do?
> ‣ What type of job do you want to be doing?
> ‣ What type of person do you need to become?

- What type of additional skills or knowledge do you need to have?

- Where do you want to go … a place or location?

- When do you want to achieve it by?

- Who is it for?

- Who will help you achieve this goal?

- Who will you involve to achieve this goal?

- Why is it important now?

- Why is it an important role for you?

Goal Defining Process

Not every question needs an answer for each goal; it is just a guide to get you started towards achieving great success. Apply this simple **Goal Defining Process** to your goals for greater clarity; complete each section of the process either as a bullet point or as a sentence …

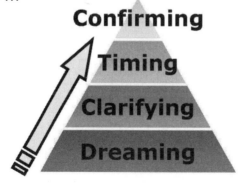

It all starts with a dream. You need to clarify an achievable realistic goal that has a timeline attached to it. Then you need to mentally confirm what it is you want to achieve.

Dreaming ...

Which area or areas does this goal relate to in your life? Please tick the appropriate boxes.

1 **Career/Business**

2 **Financial**

3 **Family**

4 **Community**

5 **Health & Fitness**

6 **Personal Growth**

7 **Adventure**

8 **Lifestyle**

List down your dream or outcome you want to achieve or the circumstances you want to change. If you knew you could be successful, (if you had no roadblocks holding you back) what could you achieve in the next 12 months in this area?

Take a moment to list your dream down ...

_____

_____

_____

_____

_____

Clarifying ...

In clarifying what you want to specifically achieve, there are most likely a number of results and feelings you will experience. Listed below are results and feelings that I have provided for you to further expand on your goal. Review the areas and ask yourself these open questions. The greater clarity of the goal, the stronger the picture you will create in your mind. Your subconscious will then identify the opportunities to pursue, plan and implement a pathway to follow.

The open questions start with ...

- Who
- When
- Where
- Why
- What
- How

In the achievement of most goals, they will have one or many of the following components, elements, feelings and results. These are just a few thought provokers to apply to the above open questions to begin the clarification of your goals.

- Size ... Big – Small – Height – Length – More - Less
- Quantity ... Number – Amount – Weight - Money
- Seen ... Visited – Colour – Shape - Image
- Quality ... Attitude – Characteristic – Knowledge - Skills
- Feeling ... Experienced – Touched - Given - Type
- Position ... Role – Title – Location - Authority
- Object ... Owned – Purchased – Obtained - Achieved

Now create a new comprehensive, in-depth, clearly defined, specific goal statement starting with ... "I have or I will or I am ..."

_____

_____

_____

Timing ...

By answering the following questions, it will assist you in establishing a timeline and a completion date in your mind. This is where the rubber meets the road. It is also the start of the confirmation part of this matrix. This is where your subconscious starts to question your beliefs and your ability to achieve this goal in this timeframe.

How much time do you need to complete this goal?

_____

When do you want to achieve it by?

_____

Why is it important now for you to achieve this goal?

_____

What is the specific day of the week, the date, the month and the year you want to achieve this goal?

_____

So from today's date, how much time is it going to take you to complete it?

_____

Can you do it in this amount of time? Circle one ... **YES** or **NO**? If it is **NO**, then adjust your timeframe, so that you can resoundingly say, **YES**!

Confirming ...

Why do you want to achieve this goal? Ask yourself this question time and time again, noting your different answers.

_____

_____

Are there any challenges that would arise if you achieved this goal?

_____

_____

What will you see when you achieve this goal?

_____

_____

What will you begin saying to yourself when you achieve this goal or what will you hear others say about you?

_____

_____

How will you feel when you achieve this goal? Have you got a clearly defined picture in your mind? Describe it.

_____

_____

Have other people achieved this type of goal before? Circle one …
YES or **NO**? Can you achieve this goal in the future if you work
your plan and plan your work? Circle one … **YES** or **NO**?

Action plan developed

I believe the reason why people don't achieve their goals is they
don't know where to start. They don't take the time to develop a
plan of action. It does not have to be a book the size of War &
Peace, but it does need to be written down.

There are three different approaches you can take that will not
only suit your personal style but even your personality. The first is
a **Detailed Plan**. It involves you looking at your specific goals and
then listing down, in no particular order, every step you think you
need to take to achieve that goal. Once you have done that, you
need to identify what order each step should be taken in. Then
identify which week or month you will take that action in and add
it to your daily or weekly planner or your To Do List for that week.

The second way is a **Chunk by Chunk** Plan. This is where you
review your goals one at a time. You will determine the first 5 steps
you need to take to get started along your journey towards the
successful completion of that goal. I know it will take more than 5
steps to achieve that goal but as you complete the five steps or
achieve each milestone, you can begin to think about the next set
of milestones or five steps.

The third is my favourite. The **Weekly Plan** involves you asking
yourself "What do I need to do this week to make that goal come
true by it's deadline?" Some goals will require no actions to be
taken and others will require a number of actions to be taken.

This plan gives you a greater degree of flexibility to adapt to your time restraints or busy schedules.

No method is better than any other; it is what suits you and your style of planning. But don't be like the majority of people who don't know where to start. They are looking for the right place to start in order to be perfect and never get started. A good friend of mine and a talented professional speaker, Malcolm McLeod, uses this quote to illustrate the point ... "A good plan started today, is better than a perfect plan started tomorrow".

Realistic time frame

You don't want to set yourself up to fail, rather give yourself every possibility of completing what you set out to achieve. To do that, you need to have realistic and believable timeframes. Timeframes that you believe you can achieve and are committed to working towards. Your timeframe needs to be like a bulls-eye. An Olympic Archer or Pistol Shooter aims at the bulls-eye of the target, not the target. The target they hit keeps them in the competition, but hitting the bull's-eye gives them the Gold Medal. Think of it this way. The outer ring is the year, then each ring going towards the bull's-eye is the month and the date.

As adults we tend to work better to a deadline. Think about the last time you went on holidays for a couple of weeks and think about your last day at work. That day you tend to be very productive. You go to work with a plan, you minimise your interruptions and you tend to be more efficient in everything you do ... phone calls, emails, meeting and paperwork. Why is it? It's because you have a deadline!

> Pursuing your passion is not about being interested or involved. It's about having a burning desire to live your dream everyday.

You know that you have to leave at 5 pm to pick up your family, collect luggage, go to the airport and catch a flight to your holiday destination. The same as you have one thing to do over the weekend around the house, but it seems to take you all weekend to do it. We work better towards a deadline otherwise it becomes the never, never plan.

Now let us reflect back on the timing section of the **Goal Defining Process**. List down the specific dates by which you want to achieve each one of your goals. At this point in time, you may start to feel very committed to your goals and that is a perfectly natural feeling to have.

> There's a big difference between interest and commitment. When you've interested in doing something, you do it when it's convenient. When you are 100% committted to your goal, you do whatever it takes to make it happen and you step out of your comfort zone.

I once had a lady come up to me at a workshop after we had completed this activity and say to me, "I feel a bit scared." My reply was "Why?" She told me that she had always set goals but never placed a deadline on when she wanted to achieve them by and now she felt very committed. A deadline made her feel more committed and in this situation, commitment is not a bad thing.

Each one of these tasks I ask you to do is a process of clarification and elimination to enhance your determination.

Get Focused

One of my personal motto's is ... **Focus on the things that count!** Believe it or not, the goal setting process is easy; the hard part is to remain focused on your goal - that is the challenge. As adults, our lives are busy, sometimes complex, maybe complicated and riddled with roadblocks. Is it any wonder that we lose focus? That's why it is critical that we continue to focus on our key goals. I love the quote ... **You will only see the obstacles when you take your eye off your goals.**

There are a number of ways to focus on your goals. Here are just a few ...

▸ **Goal Board**

- Gather pictures of your goals and put then on a cork board, wall or the refrigerator door. On your goal board, put dates on when you what to achieve the results in those pictures by. Use quotes to inspire you. I have known people who wanted to change their physical appearance, so they cut the head off the picture of a great body and put their own head on it as a goal to work towards. Do what ever it takes for you to stay focused and committed to achieving your goals.

> ### ‣ Tell a Personal Associate, your Mentors or Friends

> ▪ Share with people who are like minded and trust your goals. It is good to have someone to whom you are accountable. From time to time, they will remind you about your goal when they check on your progress. I remember when I wrote my first book I had been procrastinating.

> When two of my professional speaker buddies and I sat down to chat about our goals for the year ahead, I mentioned that I wanted to finally write my book on customer loyalty. Each of them mentioned they had a similar goal to write a book, so we started making bets on who would write their book first.

> Over the following weeks and months, we would each leave messages for one other asking how the book writing was going. It was a great wake up call to refocus myself on what my goal was. I had great delight in sending each one of them an autographed copy of my book … Creating Loyal Profitable Customers, with an invoice to remind them of them of our bet.

▸ **Review Your Goals and Your Plan**

- Once a month, sit down and review your goals. Check on your progress by acknowledging where you have been successful and identify where you need to improve your efforts.

▸ **Rewrite Your Goals**

- In order to etch your goals in your mind, rewrite your key goals every day for 30 days. This will stimulate your subconscious to be thinking about the goals that are important to you. It is a process that will assist you in creating lateral plans for your achievement.

▸ **Create a Goal Card**

- One of my favourite methods of focus is to write my goals out on a 3 x 5 card and read them every day. It is a great way to keep your goals portable. You may keep the card in your pocket or wallet or handbag or alongside your bed or on the bathroom mirror.

  The power comes from reading it every day. I can't believe the amount of people who tell me they have done that after one of my workshops. They read it every day for the year and to their surprise, achieve 8 out of the 10 goals - without even having a plan. They tell me it just seemed to happen. Nothing happens by luck; the subconscious channeled in the right direction is a powerful force to be reckoned with!

- **Meditate on Your Goals**

  - Very often, we do not take time out just to be. Once a day take 5 to 15 minutes to meditate, to have some quiet time, to get reconnected with yourself, your purpose, your passion and your goals. It is not as easy as it sounds just to stop the mind from thinking about 500 things at once.

    Just think about one goal at a time and when your mind wants to wander, refocus it on that one goal or challenge. This is a great activity to do. Just be present with yourself and be still in your thinking.

- **Electronic Reminders**

  - Some of my workshop participants have put their goals either as pictures or words on their computer as screen savers or background or on their PDA's or Mobile Phone Screens. This is probably the electronic version of a Goal Board I mentioned before. You can create your own electronic photo-album or goal card.

- **Cross Off Each Step Completed**

  - There is a magical feeling in placing a tick alongside a completed task or crossing out a milestone you have reached. If you have been working towards a saving goal, this a particularly good method. Create a picture of a thermometer and colour it in as you reach your various milestones.

It could be a calendar that you cross off as you get closer to your goal or milestone. This is a great method to use with your children and is fantastic for monitoring your progress.

▸ **Experience Your Goals**

■ Go and experience it, feel it, do it and be it for an hour or a day. Your mind needs pictures and feeling it can anchor on to. If you want to go on a holiday to Europe, go to a travel agency and collect brochures, read books and talk to people that have done what you want to do. They may even show you their photo album or videos.

If you want to buy a new car, go and test drive the one you want. Feel it. Get your photo taken with it. If you want to be employed in a certain role, go and find someone who does that and ask them about the role. I have had people who want to become a professional speakers who have followed me around for the day as I presented. People are willing to help you more than you expect. If you find someone who doesn't, find someone else.

▸ **Celebrate Your Successes**

■ If you are going to work flat out to achieve your goals and you don't celebrate it, your subconscious is going to question the reason why you are doing it.

You will find that you become bored, lethargic, unmotivated and generally lose the desire to achieve. Stop and celebrate. Life is too short to be bored and uninspired.

Enjoy your successes but don't stay celebrating for ever. Do you know people like that? They achieved sales person of the year 10 years ago and they are still dining out on it!

It does not matter where you have been, the challenges you have faced successfully or unsuccessfully. You can come back. You will need a burning desire to achieve a specific goal with a plan built upon action and an attitude that you will not be denied a positive result.

Enjoy the Journey

Don't suffer from the self inflicted epidemic of always striving but feeling like you are never arriving. In the pursuit of your goals, make sure you enjoy the journey. Don't become so obsessed with the achievement of the goal that you can't remember the journey you took to achieve your goals. It has often been said by many great authors that it is not necessarily about the goal you achieved but the person you became in the pursuit of that goal.

Here are some simple strategies to apply to your life to ensure you enjoy the journey ...

▸ Keep a journal of the milestones you achieve and the challenges you encountered along the way.

▸ Don't take yourself too seriously, laugh, have fun and enjoy the good times that you experience.

▸ Reflect on the learning experiences that you have during your journey of a lifetime.

▸ Every 3 months reflect on the past 90 days and plan ahead for the next 90 days.

Take Time to Dream Again

It is simple to always dream of the possibilities and apply the practical exercises that I have spoken about. It is about creating time and space around you to dream great dreams and to plan for their achievement. It is OK to dream! Allocate time to think about your dreams and strengthen your mental pictures of the things you want to have in your life.

The Next Step ...
Your Action Plan to Implement

- Take time to answer the goal setting questions for each of the 8 areas of your life.

- List down the specific timeframes that you will achieve each of these goals.

- List down 3 ways you are going to remain focused on your goals over the next 30 days.

- Identify 1 goal you want to achieve in the next 7 days.

Nothing is ever achieved until someone implements an idea.

Your energy may wain from time to time, but your passion will endure.

CHAPTER 4

PROGRESS
YOUR DEVELOPMENT

"It's not a revolution, it's an
evolution of your life".

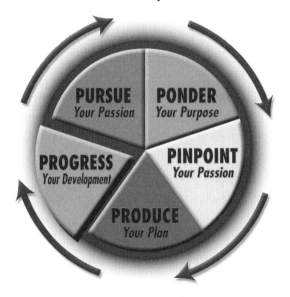

In this chapter you will discover ...

- The 8 stages of evolution, how to change before you need to change.

- Identify the 4 key areas to develop yourself personally and professionally.

- Review the 35 ways to equip yourself to achieve your true potential.

- Understand the 4 key influences in your life and how to insulate yourself from them.

Is your life evolving with the times?

If you want to progress faster towards your goals and your passion then the answer is simple … **CHANGE!!!**

I often make the comment that the reason we haven't achieved the goals we seek is that we have not changed enough to deserve them - or we have not been ready to receive them. It is like the percentage of people who win large sums of money, millions upon millions of dollars and yet two years after their windfall, they find themselves in exactly the same financial position - if not worse. They were not ready to manage the wealth they had received. They obviously did not have the right mind set nor the right attitude to deal with their situation.

To go anywhere in life, you need to grow there first in your mind. The reason you are not a millionaire is not that you don't have enough money; it is about not having a millionaire's mindset. Building wealth, managing your money and creating income producing assets are just a few key ingredients.

So think about all the goals you want to achieve in your life. Have you got the right mindset and attitude? Do you have the skills and knowledge to be the owner of your own million dollar business? What are you changing in the way you interact with your partner to create a more loving relationship? Are you changing the way you connect with your children to become a better parent? What are you doing to improve your lifestyle? What are you doing to improve your health and fitness, to tap into sustainable energy? It is about changing before you need to change!

Change is never comfortable or convenient

Most of the time, the experience of change is often perceived as an inconvenience. Change is about the choices you make and the timing of those choices. You see, I believe life is a game of either chance or choice. You chance your outcomes hoping that everything will work out for the better. You can make specific choices in your life that make a difference in the long term - or an immediate difference in the short term.

In your life, it can be beneficial that you challenge yourself by getting out of your comfort zone. Maybe this book will help you get out of the rut that you might be in at the moment. I believe your comfort zone contracts and expands during different stages of your life. As you challenge the status quo of your life, you will expand your comfort zone by altering the way you think, the way you conduct your dealings and the type of actions you take on a daily basis.

When you Choose to Change, You Become Proactive

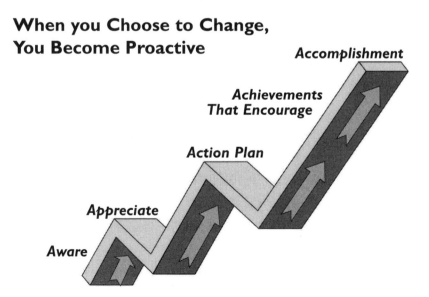

Accomplishment

Achievements
That Encourage

Action Plan

Appreciate

Aware

When you are aware you need to change, you can then truly appreciate the opportunities that arise as a result of that change. This gives you greater motivation to change for the best and implement the required action plan. With any action comes a sense of achievement. This encourages you to take the next step and then the next. Accomplishment is sure to follow.

When you Choose to Not Change, Life Becomes Reactive

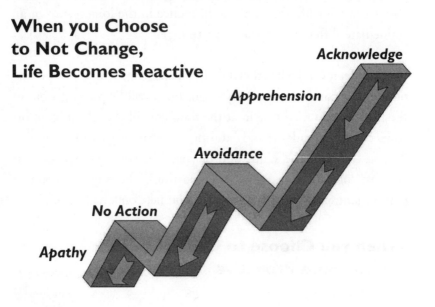

The challenge is to acknowledge your need to change. The first thing that happens is your subconscious becomes apprehensive about what might happen to you. When you step out of your comfort zone your subconscious talks you into avoiding the things that you need to do to move forward. By taking no action, you allow apathy to creep into your life, sometimes to the extent that you give up!

It starts a chain reaction. If you refuse to change the things you are not 100% satisfied with in your life, then your comfort zone will contract around you. You will choke your creative ability to dream about a better life for you and your family. It will be the ball and chain that inhibits your progress! You see, it is never the economy, your job, your partner or the school you went to that is to blame for your situation. It is all about you! You have the ability to change your attitude, your circumstances, your skill levels, your knowledge base, your mind set and your daily focus.

Change is not convenient, nor is living with mediocrity, unfulfilled dreams and untapped potential. We can only put up with mediocrity in our life because there is not enough pain to warrant us becoming uncomfortable.

On the following pages we are going to explore how best you can move yourself forward. It is about progressing yourself and your development to a level that transformation happens in your life. When this happens, you will be able to take advantage of every opportunity that comes your way. In other words you need to … **Change before you need to change!**

> # Life is meant to be an exciting journey, filled with life changing challenges, evolving experiences and memorable moments.
> # Life is about LIVING YOUR PASSION.

The 8 stages of evolution

Making changes in your life is about taking small steps that will make a difference. To do that, you will need to follow these 8 steps as you move from one place to the next in your life.

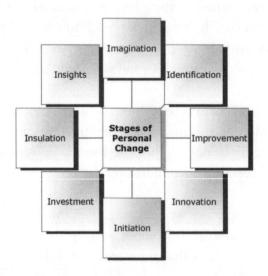

1. Imagination – Where do you want to be in the future?

2. Identification – Where are you now?

3. Improvement – What do you need to specifically do to improve?

4. Innovation – What ideas do you need to use to move forward?

5. Initiation – What are the first steps you are going to take?

6. Investment – What can you do each day to change yourself?

7. Insulation – What are the negative influences in you life?

8. Insights – What have you learnt that can shape your future?

1st Stage - Imagination …
The creator of your future

In the previous chapters of this book we have spoken about what you want to achieve in your life – both in the long term and short term. If you are going to change, then you need a reason to change - a burning desire to achieve a worthwhile goal in your life. To do that, you need to use your imagination and dream of what it would be like to be passionate, energised and enthused every day.

That is why it is critical for you to find your … **WHY!** Remember the bigger the change, the bigger the … **WHY!**

You don't need a specific reason. It can be anything at all. My reason to lose 5 kilos will be different from your reason to lose 5 kilos. You need to turn your reason into a goal. Something that gives you a positive, up-beat feel. From that goal, you will create a short term target which gives you a daily focus. This in turn strengthens your reason to change. It looks like this …

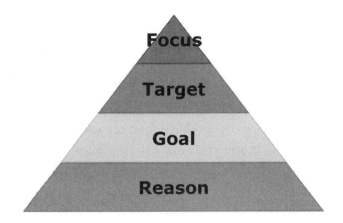

You Need a Big Reason to Change!

Your imagination needs to help play the role of creating the right goals for you to pursue. As you change who you are and what you do, your goals will change accordingly. So what do you need to change? What is your reason for changing? Use and trust your imagination. It has all the right answers!

> Our imagination needs exercise. As the saying goes, 'Use it or lose it'.

2nd Stage Identification ...
Where are you right now?

Before you move forward in anything that you do, it is important to identify the pathway you have travelled along in your life and the position you are in right now. For some people it feels like they are in a real predicament, rather than a positive place. But for each of us, life will always seem worse than it really is. We are only viewing our problems looking at it from one perspective ... ours!

Isn't it interesting that we can share our challenges with a friend or colleague? They can look at it from a different perspective, a different angle and create a simple solution for changing. But as adults, we are reluctant to humble ourselves enough to say, "I don't know how to solve it, can you show me, help me or teach me?" We need to put our ego in our pocket and ask for help. It is not a sign of weakness, but rather a sign of enlightenment! It is OK not to have all the answers.

However, you do know the answer to this question... **"Where are you right now in your life?"**

Let's determine where you are now in your life. A great analysis tool was originally introduced to me from the book called 'The Empty Raincoat' written by Charles Handy. The tool is called the **Sigmoid Curve.**

Where are you on this curve in your life, right now?

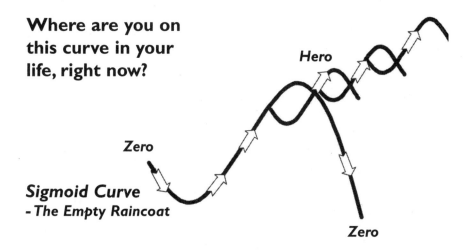

Zero

Hero

Sigmoid Curve
- *The Empty Raincoat*

Zero

You can use this tool in your personal and business life. Used on a regular basis, it can assist you in determining where you are at any given time in a number of key areas. This is purely your own personal opinion. I often refer to it as the **"Zero to Hero" Review.**

You see, we all start off in life at zero. Think about the first day on the job or when you first started out in business. In most cases, we have a number of learning experiences that are not necessarily earning experiences. We go down the hill for a period of time and then we start to master our new job in the marketplace and we work our way up to hero status in our own mind.

Then, if we don't change, we head down back to zero. That zero is normally depicted by hard times, loss of employment, loss of customers or maybe even closure of our business.

Therefore, your goal in life is to change before you need change so that you are always moving towards achieving hero status in your own life.

I think we have all known people that should have changed but didn't because they were in their comfort zone. People become complacent and don't believe they need to change because everything is going so well. You see, once we start to reach our goals, we need to be focused on the next level and to start thinking about the next set of goals, or our next achievement. This will help to avoid complacency, boredom or losing the enthusiasm for our lives.

The question highlighted on the Sigmoid Curve is relevant to your life. Ask yourself the question, "When it comes to my life, where am I right now on this curve?" Take a moment and make a mental note of where you believe you are now;

Where are you on this curve in your life, right now?

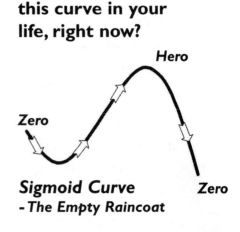

Sigmoid Curve
- The Empty Raincoat

You can use this Sigmoid Curve to map out every area of your life ...

- **Career or Business**

- **Family**

- **Finances**

- **Health and Fitness**

- **Community**

- **Personal Growth**

- **Adventure**

- **Lifestyle**

You may want to take a moment now to assess where you are situated on this curve in all of these eight areas. Be honest with yourself, but don't be too hard on yourself. I like what a good friend of mine, conference speaker Colin Pearce always says, **"You are 10 times better than what you think!"**

The good news is that it does not matter where you are on the Sigmoid Curve; it is about where you are going. This activity is about giving yourself an idea of where you feel you are positioned in life. This will determine the best way to move you forward towards personal empowerment. You need to understand the different levels of evolution.

> ## It is not what has happened to you, it's what you do that counts.

There are **5 Levels of Evolution** you will experience as you move along the Sigmoid Curve during your life. These are …

5 Levels of Evolution …

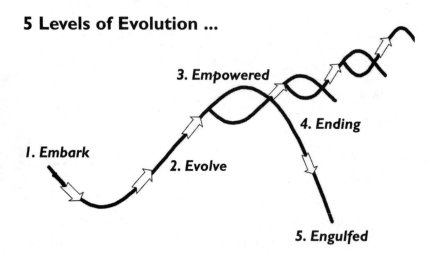

3. Empowered

4. Ending

1. Embark

2. Evolve

5. Engulfed

You will **embark** on a new journey and as you **evolve** your attitude, improve your knowledge, master your skills and increase your motivation. You will have **empowering** feelings of uncertainty about your future. However, if you don't continue to evolve yourself your successes will come to an **ending.** This means you will have departed from the habits that have helped you become empowered. If you don't change you become **engulfed** with everything in your life. It all becomes too hard. Have you felt like this or experienced this in your life?

So have you got your reason to change? Do you know where you feel you are positioned in your life? Can you start today to move yourself forward? Absolutely! It will take time and this is known as 'lag' time. There is 'lag' in time before you can reap the results from the decision to change and improve. The key is to be patient!

3rd Stage – Improvement ...
Specify what you need to improve

Kaizan is the Japanese word for continuous improvement. As adults desiring to tap into our true potential and riches that life has to offer we need to be continuously improving.

There are 4 key development components for peak performance in your life that have the greatest impact on your personal and professional growth.

> **Your Skills – The skills to complete the task.**

> **Your Knowledge – The knowledge about that subject.**

> **Your Attitude – The mind set you have about the task.**

> **Your Motivation – The desire to improve that area.**

To improve yourself it is a simple three step process that will assist you in becoming proactive in your personal and professional life.

Step 1 – Select a specific area you want to improve from the eight areas of your life.

> **Career or Business**   > **Community**

> **Family**   > **Personal Growth**

> **Finances**   > **Adventure**

> **Health and Fitness**   > **Lifestyle**

Step 2 – Clarify which **Peak Performance Development Components** need the greatest amount of attention. Give yourself a rating of between 1 and 10. On this scale 1 is the least and 10 is the most for each of the 4 components.

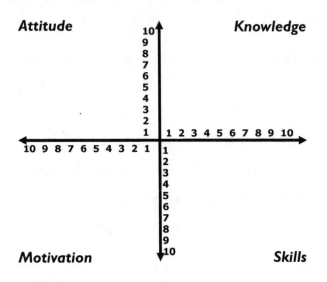

Step 3 – Then ask yourself these two questions to clarify what specifically you need to improve for you to capitalise on your potential ...

▸ **What do I do well in the ... (Specific Area)?** List down three things you do well. It is important to recognise the areas that you have mastered.

▸ **What do I need to improve in the ... (Specific Area)?** List down three things you need to improve that would assist you in moving towards your goals and overcoming any roadblocks for you to progress.

For example if you want to improve your financial circumstances in your life. Which of the 4 peak performance components are the greatest roadblocks to your future financial success? Is it a lack of skills or knowledge? Is it your attitude to your finances or do you lack the motivation to change your circumstances?

Maybe you don't have the skills on how to create a realistic budget? Maybe your mind set or attitude is focused on living for today and never planning for your future? Maybe you don't have the knowledge on how to structure your investments or you lack the motivation to stop procrastinating and making it happen.

Then ask yourself those two questions. These two steps are part of a process to clarify your action that you need to take to break through your roadblocks. This process sets you up to go to the next stage of change. Rather than ask **"Why do I need to change?"** Ask yourself, **"What do I need to change?"**

Your true passion in life will challenge your body, mind and spirit towards a triumphant achievement.

It's all in the question - what do you need to change

Here are some questions to assist you in identifying what you may need to change ...

Personal career path

‣ What do you think are the jobs, businesses and opportunities of the future?

‣ What aspects of your job do you enjoy the most? Apart from lunch time!

‣ What else would you enjoy to do as a career, a job or as a new role?

‣ What would be the perfect job or business for you in the future?

‣ What else would you like to do apart from working in your current role in your business? In other words, if you didn't work for your current business unit, what else could you do in that business or in the Marketplace?

‣ Is there an industry you would like to work in the future?

‣ Is there an opportunity in that industry now?

‣ What other businesses, companies, organisations or small business people could benefit from your skills, knowledge and talents?

‣ Who would you need to talk to that could assist you in making that transition?

‣ What would you need to do to make the transition into that type of job or role?

Personal finances

- What financial circumstances do you need to change?

- Who can you talk to that can assist you in mastering your financial circumstances?

- What books do you need to read or seminars do you need to attend to gain more knowledge about creating wealth for yourself?

- What attitudes are holding you back from becoming financially independent?

- What is your greatest roadblock to mastering your money and creating a fabulous financial future?

- What financial steps do you need to take this week to start your journey towards long term financial freedom?

- What financial plans do you have for the next 12 months, 5 years, 10 years and 20 years?

Personal relationships – Creating Great Relationships

- What are you looking for in a partner? Include qualities and characteristics.

- What aspects have you loved about some of your past relationships?

- What circumstances or situations have been repeated in your past relationships?

- What characteristics do you need to change to attract the right partner into your life?

‣ Who else in your life influences your personal relationships - family or friends or work associates?

‣ What habits, characteristics or attitudes do you need to change to create greater personal relationships in your life?

Personal relationships – Strengthening Your Relationships

‣ What can you do to enhance your existing relationships?

‣ How can you reconnect with your family and friends?

‣ Who do you need to reconnect with in your life - whether it is to mend a relationship bridge, forgive someone for a past mistake or to say "Sorry"?

‣ What have been the roadblocks for creating some close personal relationships with people?

‣ What habits, characteristics or attitudes do you need to change to strengthen your existing personal relationships in your life?

‣ Who do you need to tell that you love them and all the reasons why you love them?

Personal Fitness

‣ How do you want to look and feel everyday?

‣ What level of fitness would your like to have?

‣ What would you like to change or improve about your personal attributes?

‣ What habits do you have that stops you from achieving your fitness goals?

‣ What circumstances have you created in your life that creates roadblocks to you feeling energised on a daily basis?

‣ What is one fitness activity that you could do on a regular basis that would significantly improve your energy and fitness level?

‣ What health issues do you need to address? Whether it is going to a dentist or having a full physical by your doctor.

‣ What practises do you need to give up or start doing if you are going to live a happy, healthy, active life?

4th Stage – Innovation ...
35 Ideas to equip yourself for your future

A great author John Maxwell has an acronym for the word **EQUIP** ... **E**ncouraging **Q**ualities **U**ndeveloped **I**n **P**eople. The following ideas are suggestions, solutions and recommendations that will assist you in equipping yourself for your future. Select the ideas that are most appropriate for you right now.

1. Complete a personal review on yourself every six months

Take the time to answer these four questions as an opportunity to keep you focused and to assist in maintaining your momentum. It is a simple yet effective tool called a **W.I.S.H. Analysis.**

‣ What do you do **Well** in your personal and professional life? (Achievements)

‣ What do you need to **Improve** in your personal and professional life? (Changes)

‣ What **Strategies** do you need to develop to improve yourself? (Action)

‣ **How Long** before these strategies will be implemented into your life? (Deadline)

2. Utilise people who are close to you to give you honest feedback

You may need to take off your bullet proof vest. It is far better to obtain feedback from people who want the best for you, that you know and trust. Take their comments on board and ponder what they said, before you take any action. Have them use the W.I.S.H. Analysis so that you obtain a consistency in your feedback.

3. Establish a network of positive people around you.

Are you surrounded by people who build you up when you are down? Do they give you a positive word of encouragement? There are many negative people in the world. Make sure you have not got them all in your life. You may have family members that are negative or work associates that have a toxic attitude. It is critical that you don't become influenced by them. Love them if you must but don't let them ruin your day, week or life! Two things happen when you start to pursue your passion and develop yourself. The first is you attract other people in your life that are doing the same. The second is that people around you start to change. They are people in business and community groups who are trying to make a difference and are individuals like you who want more out of their lives.

4. Take time to rewrite your personal and professional goals.

Every three to six months, you may want to rewrite your goals. You may not want to change any of them but it is a great exercise to refocus yourself and refresh your attitude to the things that you want to achieve. There is a great deal of power in rewriting your goals. You will be amazed at the results.

Set your sights, never doubt your possibilities. Instead, doubt the limits you put on yourself.

5. Recharge your batteries

It is important that you give back time to yourself so that you can recover and recharge your energy levels. The easiest way to do that is to do the things you love to do. If you love going to the movies and getting lost in the dramatic story line, then do that. If you love playing golf with your friends, then do that. If you love taking time to have a cup of coffee and read your favourite magazine, then do that.

Do you have to do it every day, no! We tend to do things for everyone else and nothing for ourselves. Mothers are the masters at this. You can only run on empty for so long before you become emotionally bankrupt or physically exhausted. Did you know 1% of every day is 15 minutes? Do you give yourself back 15 minutes every day, just for you? You see if you don't volunteer to do this, then life will catch up with you. Fatigue, sickness and disease are the universe's way of saying, "slow down and take time off". Life has a funny way of attracting our attention.

6. Find the right mentors or coaches

Successful sporting stars like Tiger Woods who are the best in the world use a coach, then why shouldn't you? You and I need to humble ourselves enough to sit at the feet of our masters and ask them to teach us. Find the right coaches to help you to achieve your desired results. Mentors are people that are out there making things happen. Approach them, take them out for coffee and ask them for their advice and input.

There is a great deal to be learnt from people who have already blazed a pathway. When you meet, make sure you are prepared with your questions written out. This will show them that you are serious and that you are not going to waste their time.

7. Attend personal development or self improvement courses

There are numerous seminars and courses in the market place that you can attend. Identify the skills or knowledge that you need and then search the internet to find something that is in a learning format that will best suit your needs. This is an excellent way to learn as you may not have to leave your computer screen. In the back of this book there is a list of other programs that we conduct throughout the year that will enhance your personal growth and professional performance.

8. Attend company or industry related conferences

There is a great deal to be learnt when you mix with your peers. Take the opportunity to attend conferences and business seminars. Go there with the attitude that you are going to walk away with at least one good idea and that you have networked with some real movers and shakers.

The identification of your passion will help you move from an ordinary life to an extraordinary life.

9. Go back to school

You may wish to obtain some formal education by attending a University or TAFE College. This will assist you to gain the knowledge and enhance your skills. It may not be the two nights a week for the next six years, if could be one night a week for the next six weeks. One of the best courses I attended was every Tuesday night for six weeks. It was Wine Appreciation 101. It was fantastic! I was a great student, so I have had to repeat it a couple of time. I loved it. If you are learning, you are growing. Sitting in front of the TV every night will not make you a better person!

10. Listen to people who have been there and done it

If you are going to take on a new challenge, travel to a different country or enter a new career, then go and talk to people who are in that field. Organise a meeting with them and ask them some good quality questions, like …

- ‣ What has been the greatest learning experience for you when you did…(Trip, role, business)?
- ‣ What would you do differently if you were going to do it again?
- ‣ What should I do to prepare myself for this…?

- Who else should I talk to?

- What else should I do to improve my knowledge?

- What has been the highlight for you of the…?

11. Get out of your comfort zone

Do one activity a year that puts you out of your comfort zone. Ask yourself the question, "What would you find difficult to do?" Then go and do it! Maybe it is taking on a leadership role, giving a presentation to a group of peers or putting yourself in a situation where you need to meet new people. As you push your comfort zone boundaries you expand your horizons and your self confidence.

12. Improve your priority planning skills

You could choose to go and attend a time management course to learn how to prioritise your tasks, projects and organise your jobs to do. This is the difference between the people who achieve so much and the one's that wander through life. Know what steps to take to get the job done. They tend to manage their priorities rather than be consumed by their everyday tasks.

The simple approach that I personally use is to review every task I need to complete today and give it a ranking … **A – B – C.** "A" tasks are those tasks that are vital and urgent. My definition is these tasks that must be done today. "B" tasks are important but if they are not done today you won't lose a friend, your job, a customer or any money. "C" tasks are trivial; they are the nice to do if you get time. My recommendation is that you re-prioritise your list each day, if not twice a day … first thing in the morning and then after lunch as tasks present themselves.

By managing your priorities effectively you move from being out of control to being in control. Along the way you maybe from time to time having the feeling that you are adaptive ... in control, then out of control, then in control.

Moving Towards Being Proactive

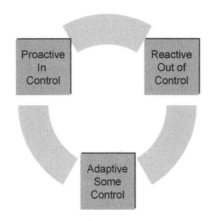

Proactive
In
Control

Reactive
Out of
Control

Adaptive
Some
Control

These are some simple techniques to manage your time, your priorities and your life ...

- ▸ **Use a diary or planner on a daily basis and group activities together – phone calls; trips to the shop; meetings.**

- ▸ **Have a big clean out and get organised. Clean out your desk; your garage; your office and your wardrobe.**

- ▸ **Look at things you can do to save minutes. Save 10 minutes each day = 36.4 hours per year.**

- ▸ **Plan today; for tomorrow and list your daily goals down.**

- ▸ **Before you say "Yes", check your priorities and schedule.**

- ▸ **Maintain a focus on the things that count for that day.**

- ▸ **Complete the toughest task first, and everything else becomes easier.**

13. List down 100 things you want to achieve in your lifetime

As I mentioned to you in a previous chapter, have some quiet time and list down your 100 goals. It will be the most insightful activity you will ever do for your personal development.

14. Join business or professional development associations

There are so many organisations and associations you can belong to. Their purpose is to provide personal and professional development to their members through a multiple of means. When you are talking to your mentors or to the people that have been there and done it, ask them which associations do they belong to or which one's would they recommend you belong to in the future.

I spent many years involved with the local cricket club, then the district cricket association. Following this I joined a local Rotaract Club, then a community based organisation that provided recreational services for disabled people. From there I joined the Brisbane Junior Chamber of Commerce and now am a member of the National Speakers Association of Australia. Every organisation along with the people I have met has been a tremendous learning experience. What could you gain from joining a community organisation?

Passionate people are not born that way, they become that way over time because of their triumphs and tragedies that they have experienced in their lives.

15. One thing you want to improve ... Work on it for 30 days

You can do anything for 30 days! You can get up early and go for a walk. You could stop eating a certain type of food. You could work for 15 minutes every day on a specific project. The esteem building power of concentrated effort will astound you. Focus your energy on creating a new habit that will change the rest of your life.

16. Readers are leaders ... Read 15-60 minutes per day

The average person reads less than one book a year. Maybe that is why they are average! If you read for 15 minutes every day you would read eight to ten books a year. If you read for 60 minutes a day then you would read a book a week - 52 books a year. What could you do with that much knowledge? How much stronger would your character be? How much more positive would your attitude become? If you want to lead yourself, then read!

17. Use the internet to your advantage

The internet is a great learning tool, so understand how to use it as a resource for your personal and professional development. Think of a topic you are interested in learning more about and go searching for an hour. Bookmark your favourite sites or subscribe to trusted information providers. We have over 6,500 people that subscribe to a weekly email called … **"The Weekly Motivator"**. To subscribe go to …
http://www.keithabraham.com.au

18. Time for a new image

Maybe it is time for a new you with a new image. Have someone give you advice on the clothes that suit you best. Maybe you need to change your hair style so that it gives you a new look. Look at the glasses you wear - maybe it is time to update your frames. Clean out the clothes you have not worn for 12 months, they are not coming back into fashion. You can't stop the aging process, but you can stop the process of looking old and outdated.

19. Understand your personality traits

The more you understand how you think and why you do things a certain way the quicker you can capitalise on your strengths and minimise your weaknesses. There are lots of different personality profiles, but the one I prefer is **DiSC Personality Profile.** You can find out more about this great personal development tool on my website – www.keithabraham.com.au under the products section.

20. Listen to audio CD's

Turn off the radio on the way to work and listen to inspirational and informational audio CD's. This is a great way to simulate your conscious and subconscious mind. Pour into your mind positive information and you will produce positive results. It is the greatest way to change your thinking. It has often been said that you need seven positive thoughts to combat one negative thought. Listening to audio CD's is great way to win the battle of possibility thinking. Go to www.livingyourpassion.com.au to see our peak performance CD's.

21. Go on retreat

When was the last time you had a weekend by yourself to totally think about yourself and your future? Take a weekend off to think about the roadmap for your future achievements without distractions. Time to plan, ponder and complete the exercises in this book. If you would find it hard to spend a whole weekend then just spend a whole day planning.

22. Face your fears

We are all fearful of something. There is a great quote from a lady called Florence Shovel Shinn, "If you face your lion on its pathway, it will dissipate". Is there one thing you need to face in your life? Maybe now is the time to stop running away from it and face it. This does not mean that you are not going to be devoid of fear from then on. It sends a message to your mind that you are stronger and not afraid of the challenges when they arrive. The longer you have carried that fear around with you, the greater the strength you will gain from it - when you face it.

23. Take a break from your normal routine

During our lifetime we all get into routines and that is fine, except when it turns into a rut. Break some limiting patterns in your life. Go to work a different way. Instead of holidaying in the same spot all the time visit a different place. Eat at different restaurants. Pursue a different past time. Break the routine; you can always revert back to it later if you wish. Who knows you may enjoy different experiences and a whole new world waiting for you.

24. Complete a speed reading course

If readers are leaders, then learning how to read faster and more effectively is going to assist you in making your personal and professional development transition. You can do this type of course over a weekend at TAFE Colleges all around the country. Maybe take the time to explore some different courses at the same time.

25. Conquer procrastination

There is a funny poem about procrastination. It goes like this ...

> *Procrastination is my sin.*
> *It brings me endless sorrow.*
> *I really must do something about it.*
> *In fact I will start tomorrow.*

Start today! Do you suffer from procrastination? Do you put things off? I believe procrastination is the greatest robber of self esteem! If you know you should do something and you don't do it, then that eats away at your self esteem. On the other hand self discipline is the greatest enhancer of self esteem.

To beat procrastination, it is a simple process. First identify the task you have been procrastinating about and then determine the first simple step you must do in order to tackle that task. Set a time and a date to do it. If you do not have a good track record when it comes to starting projects!

Here are the simple questions that you can follow ...

- **What are you procrastinating about in your life?**
- **How long have you been procrastinating about these tasks, jobs or activities?**
- **How long would it take you to complete this task?**
- **What would be the first step you could take to start this task?**
- **When could you start that first step and when could you finish it by? Think about the day, date and time.**
- **What is stopping you from starting?**

At this point of time you need to make one of two choices. Do you complete the task and get it over and done with, or if you don't do it – you must be prepared to suffer the consequences. You always have the choice. If you need to complete the task you have been procrastinating about, then stop beating yourself up and just do it!

As the people at Nike would say ... Just Do It! I was looking through a T-shirt shop during one of my trips and saw a t-shirt that had the famous Nike Tick reversed. Instead of **Nike,** it had **Pike.** The slogan underneath it was ... Just Didn't Do It. Don't pike out on your life, beat procrastination and just do it!

As the sun comes up in the day and the stars fill our skies, passionate people will always achieve great things.
This is a universal law.

Life and time waits for no one as this next verse demonstrates!

To realise the value of one year:
Ask a student who has failed a final exam.
To realise the value of one month:
Ask a mother who has given birth to a premature baby.
To realise the value of one week:
Ask an editor of a weekly newspaper.
To realise the value of one hour:
Ask the lovers who are waiting to meet.
To realise the value of one minute:
Ask the person who has missed the train, bus or plane.
To realise the value of one second:
Ask a person who has survived an accident.
To realise the value of one millisecond:
Ask the person who has won a silver medal in the Olympics.

26. Participate in community service work

This is always a great lift in your self esteem and self confidence when you help other people achieve and when there is no direct benefit to you. Many years ago I was involved in a Rotaract Club. Rotaract is a youth project sponsored by Rotary International. They are a group of people aged 18 to 30 with the purpose of developing themselves by helping people through service to the community.

We worked on many great projects from planting trees; car washes; hosting a world conference of Rotaractors, all to raise hundreds of thousands of dollars for the community. The most memorable project of all which has stuck with me for almost 20 years, was a community service activity called ... Rent–A–Santa. It is where the Rotaractors would pair up and we would get dressed up as Santa and his helper. We would visit families on Christmas Eve delivering presents to families who wanted their children to have an extra special Christmas treat.

A fellow Rotaractor Margot Wright and I were asked to visit this one family in Ashmore, Gold Coast, Queensland. Now normally the family would leave some presents out for us near the letterbox so that we could put them in Santa's Sack and give to the young children once we were inside the house.

It was always an amazing feeling with the children getting really excited to see Santa. At this particular house there were no presents. We always carried some extra gifts in the car so we took those inside. When we arrived there were no presents under the Christmas tree and the single mother had her hands in her head at the kitchen table.

This family had fallen on some tough times and couldn't afford Christmas presents. The look of gratitude in that Mother's eyes knowing her children were going to have the joy of Christmas has stuck with me forever. It still brings a tear to my eye.

There is magic in helping other people that warms your own heart, and touches your soul. It is not until you have taken your eyes off yourself that you can truly appreciate the gifts that we have been given in life.

Do you have to join a club to do this – of course not! It could be to raise money for a special cause or charity with your work colleagues. You may help a next door neighbour out. It could be you assist in organising a High School Reunion. There are many things that you can do for others. Open your eyes and your heart will follow.

27. Meditation and being still

Being present with yourself is a powerful tool in controlling your thoughts. Through meditation and being still is a great way to focus your mind. We live in a fast paced action packed world. Find a quiet place for 15 minutes at least once a day and just be still, slow down your mind, breath and smell the roses. This is a great way to reconnect with your higher purpose and either prepare for the day ahead or relax from the day you have just had.

28. Create your own mastermind group

There is a great deal of power created when a group of like minded people get together to share ideas, learning experiences and uncommon wisdom. I am in a Mastermind Group with four other professional speakers that I come together with every two months. We share ideas, projects we are working on and we use each other as a sounding board. Think about creating your own group of people where you get together once every three months for a lunch or breakfast. To make this effective operate under some basic rules and principles and have a set agenda.

Here is a suggested format as your agenda to get you started ...

- ‣ Welcome
- ‣ Wins that people have had in the past three months
- ‣ Challenges encountered – suggestions provided
- ‣ Assistance needed
- ‣ Future goals and projects for the next three months
- ‣ Date for next mastermind meeting and coordinator

29. Create a positive networking group

Following on from the Mastermind Group concept - you can create your own networking group where you organise a larger group of people. You then become the conduit that brings people together so that they can connect with like minded people. Whether this group has a business focus or a social focus is up to you. If you want to surround yourself with positive people what better way to do it than by creating your own network of positive people. If you purchase the book ... **Networking to Win** by Robyn Henderson, she gives some great tips on how to do this. See her book review at www.keithabraham.com.au/articles.php

30. Week long focus

If you want to learn a new skill or to rekindle an interest in an old hobby then organise to spend a week doing it. It might be a golf school, cooking class, wine appreciation, fishing trip, art classes or business retreat. Concentrating your efforts not only builds your enthusiasm for your interest but perfects your skills.

31. Write a book

Mark Victor Hansen the co-author of Chicken Soup for the Soul Series and the One Minute Millionaire book, once said to me that there is million dollar best selling book inside everyone. It is an enlightening and evolving experience to write about something you are passionate about. It might be a history of your family, a children's book, a fable, a mystery novel, a "How to ..." book or a short story. It could be 10 pages or 1000. The process of writing helps us to learn, understand, accept and heal.

If you feel there is author inside of you visit my website ... www.pursuingyourpassion.com so that you can find out more how you can write and sell your book.

32. Deliver a presentation

It is often said if you want to learn something, go and teach it. The best way to do that is through a presentation. There are organisations like Toastmasters International and Rostrum that will teach you how to speak. Once again you may like it so much you want to do it as a business. Visit my website. We have great tools and articles for you to start down the path of your professional speaking career.

> **People don't care what has happened to you, they want to know what you're going to do with what's happened to you.**

33. Relive a childhood dream or adventure

Have you ever gone back to your old neighbourhood where you grew up and mentally relived some of your adventures and recalled some of your learning experiences? For most of us some of our childhood memories are some of our fondest. This activity also helps us to recall some of our childhood dreams. The things we were going to do when we grew up. Why don't you relive the past and rekindle the passions that you had, all over again.

34. Doing nothing

There is also a time and a place to do nothing. Our lives can be hectic and out of control. Maybe it is time for you to stop and take control of what matters most to you. How would you feel if you scheduled in your diary to do nothing at all for one whole day, for a weekend or for a week. Refresh yourself!

35. Take a sabbatical

There is a great book written, Time off from work: Using sabbaticals to enhance your life while keeping your career on track by Lisa Rogak. It shares some great ideas on how to create the situation in your life to have a sabbatical. You may need to take your long service leave to fall back in love with your career or business or life. It could be time to reinvent who you are and what you do. Maybe it is only for a one or two months. Maybe you could travel around the country or swap homes with someone overseas or pursue your passion for a couple of months on a fulltime basis.

5th Stage – Initiation …
Taking small steps

With the 35 ideas that I have given you, to inspire you and think about, you now have enough material to formulate a specific self development strategy for the next 3 - 6 - 9 months. It may not be about creating dramatic changes in your life but moving yourself from ordinary to dynamic.

In 1956 Melbourne hosted the Olympics, a young man named Murray Rose won the Gold Medal for the 1500 metres freestyle swimming event. In 2000, Sydney played host to the XXVII Olympiad and another young man Grant Hackett won the Gold Medal for the 1500 metres freestyle swimming event. If we could have wound back time and had Grant Hackett to race against Murray Rose, Grant Hackett would have beaten Murray Rose by more than six laps of an Olympic Pool. Yes pools have gotten quicker, swim suits have gotten longer, training techniques and schedules have improved, but no one ever said that we are going to shave a lap off the time this year. They focused on half a second and continuously improved over a 44 year period.

Changes are made one step at a time, 1% at a time and by taking small steps on a regular basis. Make changes this week that have an impact on next week, and make changes next month that have an impact on the following month. So what are you going to do in the next 30 – 60 – 90 days to progress yourself towards a higher self esteem, self confidence and self belief? Identify three things that you could do over the next 90 days that would have a greater impact on your life.

> ## Your best investment, is the one you make in yourself!

Take a moment to look at an example of a self development schedule ...

Sample of a yearly self development schedule

January	Read 1 personal growth book
February	Set up a mastermind group
March	Select a course to attend at TAFE
April	Spend time reviewing my goals
May	Find a career mentor to meet
June	Have my second mastermind meeting
July	Join an Industry based Association
August	Spend time reviewing my goals
September	Read 1 personal growth book
October	Have my third mastermind meeting
November	Attend a meditation course
December	Start planning next year's goals

The power of your passion will pull you towards your desires and destinations.

6th Stage – Investment …
Doing something every day

There is an old affirmation, "Every day in every way I get better and better." Developing yourself is a do it to yourself every day project. It is not about being consistently inconsistent. It is about doing little things every day to keep the momentum happening in your life and ensuring that you become better and better every day.

One concept that you may want to think about is to create the perfect day to enhance your progress. What could you do each day that would make you feel great about yourself and that would assist you in combating the negative influences that you may have had in your life?

Here are some of the activities that work for me on a daily basis …

- I read my goal card with my goals written down for the year.
- I exercise for 15 – 60 minutes.
- I eat a healthy breakfast.
- I read my affirmations.
- I eat a balanced healthy diet with few, if any treats.
- I read a personal development, business or autobiography book for 15 – 60 minutes.
- I tell my wife and children I love them.
- I start the day with a goal and a prioritised plan of action.
- I send a note or an unconditional gift to someone as a thank you.

Remember, if you don't invest in yourself, whether that be time or money, why would anyone else invest in you?

Do I do all of these things every day. Not all of them but the majority of them every day. These activities keep me focused and assist me in maintaining a positive, can do attitude.

What are you going to do to maintain your positive attitude every day? It is always the little things that make the biggest difference in your life. Think about five things you can today that would lift your self esteem, enhance your self confidence and give you greater belief in your ability to achieve.

1. _____

2. _____

3. _____

4. _____

5. _____

When you are a passionate person and have a purpose, you have a presence that draws opportunities to you.

7th Stage – Insulation …
Protect yourself from negative influences

We are influenced by a number of factors. It is what is happening in our sphere of influence and especially what is happening in our minds.

Influencing Factors

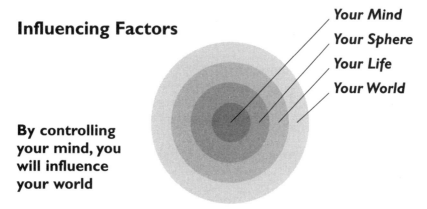

Your Mind
Your Sphere
Your Life
Your World

By controlling your mind, you will influence your world

The more we move ourselves from the inside to the outside, the less influence we have over the circumstances. However, if you can control your mind, influence your thought patterns and maintain a positive perspective on your attitude you will change your world.

Each of us become plugged in and emotionally engaged when our buttons are pushed - whether it is from someone making an off handed comment about our work or family. It might bring up something that you did 20 years ago, that you were not proud of doing.

It is OK to get upset as long as it does not disable you from functioning effectively and rationally. If this happens to you, you are giving away all of your personal power that controls how you think, which in turns effects the way you act. Remember your actions will speak louder than words.

There are a number of areas that will have the biggest impact in assisting you to take control, gaining greater personal power and enhancing your presence. These four areas are the roadblocks that stop people from changing and moving forward.

- ‣ Personal Circumstances
- ‣ Personal Attitudes
- ‣ Personal Beliefs
- ‣ Personal Actions

Personal circumstances

Don't stay in a situation you don't like. Either change the situation or change your attitude to that situation. If there are friends that bring you down and dump on you, don't spend time with them. If there is something you don't like fix it or forget about it. It is important that you keep your focus in the present time, learn from the past, plan for the future and live for the present moment. Make sure you are willing to laugh at yourself, at life and with others. Life is too short not to, so don't take yourself so seriously.

Personal attitudes

Your attitude determines where you will go in your life. People with wonderful attitudes have great lives. Start to generate positive thoughts and feeling about yourself. Replace your thoughts of inadequacy with ones that you can achieve. Be in charge of your thoughts!!!

Personal beliefs

Do you think about positive results or all the negative things that will happen to you? Be your best friend not your worst enemy. Avoid comparing yourself to others! Accept other people's acknowledgements and compliments.

Personal actions

Activity cures inactivity! In other words stop talking about it and take action. You cannot steer a parked car, it needs to be moving. So take any action to get started, don't wait for the circumstances to be perfect. Become accountable for the results your actions produce. Be assertive, speak up for yourself.

Learn to communicate openly, ask for what you want. Remember the answer is always no, if you don't ask the question! Take every opportunity to do something for others and acknowledge others frequently. Tell them what you like and appreciate about them (especially your family, partners and work associates).

> In living your passion you are only limited by your level of belief in what you can achieve.

8th Stage – Insights ...
Looking back to move forward

It is the recognised insights that make us wise. Everyday there is something that can be learnt. My cousin has an inquisitive young boy Connor, who is 5. His dad was putting him to bed one night he seemed a bit sad and my cousin asked, "What was wrong?" He replied in a disappointed way, "I didn't learn anything new today".

If we stop learning then that is when we stop growing as people. We can learn from everyday and every person, only if we tune our awareness into learning. Take time each day to reflect on the day, your flashes of brilliance, your learning opportunities and what you will do different next time. Remember you will become insane, if you keep on making the same mistake over and over again and not learning from them.

Start to keep a journal alongside your bed and jot down your insights from the day or week and recognise the wonderful things you do and identify the things you would do differently next time, given the opportunity.

You may not see the steps you need to take to transform your life, however by taking small steps every day you will change and evolve. It is like the story of this rare Bamboo Plant, you have to water it for 5 years before it shoots up from the ground. Now that takes a great deal of faith. But in the 5 year, it grows 20 metres in 5 weeks.

Have faith in yourself and make small steps every day to growing and developing yourself. You will never make a greater investment!

To know true triumph, you must
first have a passion.

The Next Step ...
Your Action Plan to Implement

- Take time to complete the 'change' questions in all the key areas of career, finance, fitness, and relationships. Use your personal journal or notebook to list your answers down.

- Complete the W.I.S.H. Analysis Activity.

- Identify 5 activities you are going to undertake in the next 90 days that will aid you in your personal and professional growth.

- Identify the one task you have been procrastinating about doing and complete it in the next 7 days.

Having goals won't make you passionate, but taking great actions will set you on a pathway towards becoming a passionate person.

Be inspired by your desire, fuelled by your actions, powered by passions and satisfied by your success.

CHAPTER 5

PURSUE YOUR PASSION

"Let's begin the journey".

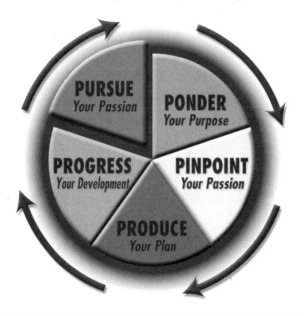

In this chapter you will discover ...

- It is not about what has happened in the past, it is what you are going to do in the future that counts.

- Overcoming the tests along the way towards reaching your goals.

- Identify the 12 ways to magnetise your mind set in order to be open to creating a great life for yourself.

- Understand that it is your choice to achieve great things in your life.

Are you ready for the journey called … "Your Life!"

Your life is a journey. How exciting it is and how passionate a pursuit it becomes is up to you. Like any journey, there are a number of components that will assist you in pursuing your passion as you move forward. The following are elements I believe will aid you in your journey towards reaching your passions. With these elements as your focus, you can conquer the challenges you will encounter along the way. They will help you create momentum in your pursuit and keep you focused on enjoying the journey.

They say that if you want to stop a train from moving, then you should place a wooden chock in front of it. It won't move, even with the engine engaged and acceleration applied. Why? It has no momentum to move itself over the wheel chock. However, if that same train is travelling 50 kilometres an hour, then 3 metres of a reinforced concrete wall would not stop its momentum.

Regardless of the size of steps you take, any action will start to create momentum in your life. If I had a choice between being motivated and having momentum in my life, momentum would be my first choice every time. With momentum behind you, you can achieve anything. The challenges you face will become milestones you will have conquered along your journey.

> # Your victories are hollow if you have never known disappointment.

Forget the past – focus on your future

Now more than ever before, you need to draw a line in the sand and forget about what has happened to you in the past. You need to focus on following the pathway to your passions. As adults, we tend to focus too much on our past challenges. Don't let your past dictate your future. Your future is bright, brilliant and buoyant.

In 1954, Roger Bannister broke the 4 minute mile. What is amazing about Bannister's story is the journey he had taken to achieve his goal. You see, Bannister had to earn the respect of his peers at Oxford University for a year by cleaning up after them and shovelling snow before he was allowed to compete in their track and field team. When he did, he was fast, fluid and stood out amongst the other team members. Catching the eye of the Great Britain track and field Olympic selectors, he was selected to represent his country at the 1952 Helsinki Olympics and with that selection rode the gold medal hopes of all of Great Britain.

He made the final of the 1500 metres race and when the final bell rang, he gave his famous kick for the last lap. Simultaneously, many of his fellow competitors shifted gear and in the end Bannister didn't get a place. In some of the London newspapers, the headline read 'Bannister Fails!' He felt he had let down his country, his university and himself. Like all great achievers Bannister knew the key was not how far you fall, but how you bounce back that counts.

He set a goal that he would redeem himself and break the four minute mile barrier. This was a goal that many believed was physically impossible. Other athletes had been attempting to achieve the same goal for the past nine years.

With his medical background and knowledge of athletics, he planned his attack. He researched mechanical aspects of running and developed a scientific training method to aid him. At Iffley Road, Bannister planned to have two runners, Chris Brasher and Chris Chataway, to pace him for his attempt on breaking the 4 minute mile. The weather on the day was horrible, with 15mph crosswinds gusting up to 25mph, and Bannister very nearly called the attempt off. Despite the poor weather, a large crowd gathered to fill the stands and support Bannister's attempt.

When the race started, Chris Brasher took the lead as the first pacemaker. Bannister slotted in behind him, with Chataway in third place. When Brasher began to tire, Bannister gave the signal for Chataway to take over. The officials rang the bell to indicate the last lap and the crowd started clapping. With just over two hundred yards to go to the finish, Roger Bannister took the lead and kicked with the crowd now standing and cheering him on. He sprinted to the line and finishing in a time of 3:58.4. He had done it. He had come back!

When he was asked to explain that first four-minute mile—and the art of record breaking—he answered with original directness, **"It's the ability to take more out of yourself than you've got."**

Set your sights, never doubt your possibilities. Instead, doubt the limits you put on yourself.

> You can come back. You just need a
> bigger reason why, rather than why not.

Decide to go on your journey now!

If it is not now - then when? Make the decision to follow your passions and pursue your dreams. Stop wondering if it is going to be the right thing to do. Let me tell you, you will never make the wrong decision. Every decision you make is 100% correct, for that time and place.

A day later, a week later or a year later it may not have been the right decision. So change it, fix it, make it right and move on! Don't procrastinate and shift into a permanent pause mode. Everything that you have read about in this book is about following simple processes and formulas that will assist you in clarifying your goals. Part of the process is to motivate yourself to obtain 100% commitment for the goals you have set. As you follow the process, you will know in your heart of hearts if that is the right goal for you to pursue at that time.

Your roadmap is your planned pathway

With a plan, all things are possible. You would not jump in a commercial airliner not knowing what destination you wanted to end up arriving at, would you? So why go through life or try to achieve your goals without a plan? Your roadmap does not have to be planned out in its entirety. Plan a month in advance if that suits your style and be willing to have flexibility. Just be clear on your final destinations and milestones that you want to achieve along the way. It is critical that you start today. What is one thing that you can do today to start? It may only take you five minutes to do it. Don't delay start today!

Remember there are many different pathways to your goals. If one pathway is blocked, then try an alternate route. Go cross country if you must; blaze your own pathway so that others can follow you.

> Believe the plan will work for you and know it will need work from you!

You will be tested with challenges

There will be challenges and roadblocks along the way. They have been put there to test your desire to achieve that goal and your resolve to obtain your passion. From my experience, life will always test you as soon as you set a goal. Take weight loss for example, and imagine you want to lose 5 kilos for summer. You set the goal, you have a plan and you're ready to start Monday morning.

That is the day that it rains just as you are about to go for your walk. That is the day that someone brings in homemade chocolate cake - just like your Mum used to make. It is all a test!

It happens doesn't it? A very good friend of mine, James Kennett had a great saying, "Forewarned is forearmed". You have been warned, so now be prepared for it. Whinging and whining won't get the job done. Don't consider your challenges as problems, but as opportunities to strengthen your character. It is all about how you look at it.

What do you see?
OPPORTUNITYISNOWHERE
Or
OPPORTUNITY/IS/NOW/HERE

Magnetising your mind set

Your mind set and attitude are one of the greatest attractors of good things coming into your life. A poor mindset can also be the one thing that pushes great opportunities away from you. The following are simple thoughts to focus on in order to magnetise your mindset ...

1. **Take full responsibility for your life** – Become accountable for the results your actions produce. Don't lay blame on others to justify the circumstances of your life.

2. **Generate positive thoughts and feelings** – Replace your old thoughts of inferiority and inadequacy. Be in charge of your thoughts. If you can control your mind, you can control your world.

3. **Do things you like to do** – Don't stay in a situation you don't like. Either change the situation or change your attitude towards it. Life is too short to be feeling out of control!

4. **Watch what you say to yourself** – Avoid self put-downs and being critical of yourself. It is now time to be your best friend - not your worst enemy.

5. **Keep your focus in the present** – Learn from your past, plan for your future and live for the present. Remember life is to be lived, experienced and enjoyed.

6. **Accept other people's acknowledgements and compliments** – Don't invalidate other people's positive thoughts and feelings about you. Just say **'Thank you'** and let yourself enjoy them without embarrassment rather than getting into a debate about what the other person said to you.

7. **Avoid comparing yourself to others** – See yourself as being of equal worth. Remember, our value as human beings is not derived from what we do; it comes from who we have become.

8. **Whenever you have a thought that starts with "I have to ... I ought to ... I need to ... I should ... I'd better"** – Change it to "I want to or I choose to". By doing this, you become in charge of your thoughts, not controlled by them.

9. **Be willing to laugh at yourself, at life and with others** – Stop taking yourself so seriously. If you make a mistake, get over it, forgive yourself and treat it as a learning experience.

10. **Acknowledge others frequently** – Tell people close to you what you like and appreciate about them – including your family, partners and work associates.

11. **Be assertive, speak up for yourself** – Learn to communicate openly, ask for what you want, express and share your feelings, preferences and opinions openly and without fear.

12. **Take every opportunity to do something for others** – Freely allow others to do things for you.

What are you going to pack for your journey?

Leave home with the right attitude - it is going to be fun. It is not just about striving to reach your goal, it is also about arriving at your destination a better person than when you began. Stop and enjoy the moments and the marvellous milestones you achieve along the way. Celebrate your successes! This is the way to recharge your batteries to continue on with your journey.

You will need to understand that tenacity wins every race. It is not how fast or how slow, it is about how you grow during the experience. I often say you need to grow there mentally before you will go there physically.

Pack a willingness to make it happen for yourself. No one else can do it for you. It is your responsibility to design a life you want to live, to take small steps to create momentum in your life towards your goals and passions. You see, once you have momentum then you can become unstoppable! You will become passionate about your life and about your goals.

What's Your Premonition?

I have a premonition that soars on silver wings.

I dream of your accomplishments and other wondrous things.

I do not know beneath what sky or where you will challenge faith.

I only know it will be high.

I only know you will be great.

Before You Start Your Journey

It is your choice. You may have questions going through your mind like, Why Me? Why Now? The questions I have for you are simply; Why not you? Why not right now? Are you going to be someone who goes through the motions? Are you someone who just gets by? Are you going to be good at what you do? Are you able to realise your full potential? Are you going to be someone that is great at what they do in their life? I wish you success in your journey towards living your passions.

It is Your Choice

You can walk in the valleys, but I'm not coming too,

Because I will be out there climbing mountains, where you can see the view.

You can look through an atlas, and see the world from afar,

But I would rather you be out there reaching to catch a shooting star.

You can lie there watching the best of your life go by,

But wouldn't you rather be out there dancing on a hill where eagles fly.

You can sit in the shadows, wishing you could see,

But wouldn't you rather be out there achieving, what ever you want to be.

And if you want the secret of how to win or lose,

Then listen and I'll tell you – all you do is choose!

The Next Step ...
Your Action Plan to Implement

- **What is one action step you can take in the next 60 minutes to make some progress towards one of your goals?**

- **What are you going to do in the next 24 hours to take one positive step towards your desired outcomes?**

- **What are you going to do in the next 7 days to work towards you high priority goals?**

Learn from hindsight, to gain insights to improve your foresight.

Great things are all around us,
but greatness is within us.

Final Message

Well done! You have achieved the first milestone of your journey by finishing this book. You are now in the top 30% of people. You see, only 30% of books purchased are ever read and of that 30%, only 40% of people ever get past chapter 3. So congratulate yourself on taking the time to invest in your future.

To assist you in remaining focused, I have created an oasis of positive resources for you at my website ... www.livingyourpassion.com.au On this website you will find numerous ways to recharge your batteries through positive weekly quotes, online coaching programs, articles and support materials.

My goal for you is that you realise your potential, rise up above your current challenges and make claim to your future. Take the opportunity to tap into your greatest asset. You deserve adventure, financial security, good health, love, success and most of all, happiness. I wish you the very best of everything life has to offer - because you deserve it all.

I trust that 'Living Your Passion' has provoked you, inspired you and made a difference in your life.

Sincere regards,

Keith Abraham

Passionate Stories Wanted

I don't know about you, but I draw a great deal of strength from people who are out there making a positive difference in their own lives. If that is you, then I would love to hear your story.

Would you like to be a star in one of my next books? Tell me about how you have applied the principles and processes from this book into you day to day lives. Tell me how it has changed your mind set or focus and what you have achieved.

We all have a story to tell. Regardless of how small an achievement it may seem to you, I have no doubt that it will give the people who read it HOPE. Even if you don't want me to share it with anyone else, I would still love to here it. A lady once wrote to me after attending our 1 day **"Living Your Passion" Workshop** telling me that she went home and for the first time set goals with her husband after 22 years of marriage. They virtually changed their whole lives over night. They were in jobs they both hated and lived an existence of quiet desperation. Her email really moved me and just continues to reinforce the power of goal setting.

So here is the deal, if you send your success story to keith@livingyourpassion.com.au then I will send to you a free e-book manual called "Reconnecting with Your Passion, Family and Yourself." I look forward to reading your story.

About the Author

Keith Abraham

Ninety-Seven percent of people have few or no goals. Keith has spent half of his life researching the goal setting process and defining what it takes to be your own motivator, discover your own passions in life and get paid to do what you love. Keith's ideas, insights and passion have touched over 300 000 people in the 8 years he has been presenting on peak professional and personal performance. Keith guarantees to give you a step by step action plan and the how to's on living your passion.

About Keith's Keynotes, Workshop Topics and Customised Training

> ‣ *Customer loyalty;*
> *How to create loyal profitable customers Marketing*
> *Business growth » Service experience » Customer loyalty*

> ‣ *People motivation;*
> *How to pursue your passion and design a life worth living*
> *Motivation » Inspiration » Confidence » Direction*

> ‣ *Sales performance;*
> *How to maximise and optimise your selling opportunities*
> *Sales direction » Optimise opportunities » Classify customers »*
> *Maximise marketing efforts*

> ‣ *Conquering change;*
> *How to change, challenge and conquer your marketplace*
> *Evolving your business » Innovative ways to change*
> *» Challenging marketplace mediocrity » Change before you*
> *need to change*

Results speak…

"The conference workshop was extremely successful and the feedback received has exceeded all expectations. Keith is an exceptional speaker who is able to motivate and capture his audiences using a variety of innovative styles and methods."

Judy Fenton, Human Resources Manager Collins Foods International.

"Your presentation at Langkawi was filled with humour, facts and logic."

Ian Davison, Country Advertising Agency

"Feedback from these meetings has been the best ever. Your segment was spot on for the target audience."

Alan Porich, Divisional General Manager, Toyota Australia

To have Keith speak at your next conference or design a customised training package for your organisation, visit our website, www.keithabraham.com.au or email keith@keithabraham.com.au

Peak Personal and Professional Passion CD Series

Passion for Customer Loyalty CD Series

How to create loyal, profitable customers

You will discover how to develop a contact strategy program to ensure frequent customer interaction – so you remain top of mind. You will understand the time-proven methods that support your customer's buying decisions after the selling transaction by using the 55 loyalty gaining ideas. You will be able to identify why customers give you their loyalty and why others will never be loyal to your brand or products. **RRP $319.** To order, visit our website www.livingyourpassion.com.au

Passion for Prospecting CD Series

How to create an endless supply of prospects eager to purchase your products.

What you will discover is how to create a business profile in your market place that will attract prospects eager to do business with you. You will be given specific strategies on how to gain rivers of referrals and an endless supply of qualified prospects for your business. **RRP $147.** To order, visit our website www.livingyourpassion.com.au

Passion for Customer Service CD Series

How to create a world class customer service experience in your business.

You will discover the 10 critical success factors that lay the foundation for an exceptional customer service experience in your business. You will learn how to influence your customer's buying decision and buying motives in your market. We will review the time-proven strategies for customer service success in 4 key areas and understand how to initiate a quality control system to ensure a consistent customer service experience is delivered. **RRP $319.** To order, visit our website www.livingyourpassion.com.au

Passion for Selling CD Series

How to sell any product to anyone in any market place.

You will discover the secrets of the Top 1% of Sales Professionals and how they use them to exceed there sales budget every year. These time-proven selling strategies and ideas will enable you to double or triple your income. You will be amazed at the results you will achieve to become significant in your market place. **RRP $319.** To order, visit our website www.livingyourpassion.com.au

Peak Personal and Professional Passion CD Series cont...

Passion for Presentation Skills CD Series

How to present with Power, Pizzazz and Poise.

You will discover a simple 3 part model on how to construct a polished presentation that engages your audience and influences them in positive and powerful ways. You will understand what skills are required to make your presentation a 'work of art' that will have your audiences wanting more. You will learn how to use PowerPoint to get your point across and how to make any material interesting without detracting from you being the star of the show. **RRP $319** To order, visit our website www.livingyourpassion.com.au

Passion for Marketing CD Series

How to create 21 compelling reasons to do business with you.

You will gain a clear understanding of how to identify and combine your Unique Selling Proposition, Visual Selling Proposition and Emotional Selling Proposition to provide a compelling reason to do business with you. You will discover how to build your brand, your personal and business presence using little or no capital. **RRP $319.** To order, visit our website www.livingyourpassion.com.au

Passion for Business Development CD Series

How to optimise and maximise your existing client base to increase your bottom line.

You will discover how to build customer relationships that stand the test of time using 55 time proven contact strategies. You will learn how to implement low cost and no cost strategies to gain your customer's loyalty. You will learn how to take 5 simple steps that will evolve your business to take advantage of your current business opportunities. Also, you will review the 6 secrets to maximising your business profits. **RRP $319** To order, visit our website www.livingyourpassion.com.au

Passion for Leadership CD Series

What you will discover.

The Keys to Working Together as One Team with a Common Purpose; Defining the Priority Goals and Organisational Direction; Building Your Team Relationships in Order to Achieve Your Strategic Plans; Developing a Charter on How you Work Together as Leadership Committee; How to Work Smarter with Greater Productivity as a Senior Management; A Review of the Leadership Team's - Strengths and Weaknesses; Develop Your Strategic Business Plans and Define Your Team Projects. **RRP $147.** To order visit our website www.livingyourpassion.com.au

If you absolutely loved Keith's book, and you want to know how you can truly live your passion ... this is an event you won't want to miss!!

Join us at the Living Your Passion seminar and learn Keith's 5 simple steps to living a life filled with Success, Wealth and Achievement.

Frustrated with how much (or how little) you earn? Hate your current job or business? Love to be earning a great living doing something you absolutely love doing?

☐ Do you want to have more success and wealth in your life?

☐ Would you like to achieve all of your wildest dreams?

☐ Do you ever feel like everyone else is getting ahead?

☐ Have you ever failed and never knew why?

☐ Do you want to know how to get more your relationships and your life?

☐ Would you like to know how to turn set backs into stepping stones towards true personal success?

If you can answer YES to any of these questions this event is a "must".

Max Walker says Keith's life is an extension of his passion ...

"I share the stage with a great variety of presenters –
informative, inspirational, humourous and technical.
When Keith is on the programme I know it's going to be a
stimulating session for he embodies all of the above. I admire
people pursuing their dreams with passion. Keith's life is an
extension of his passion and his presentations make both an
impact and a difference. His value add and take away elements
are uncomplicated and can be used immediately by the
business groups he shares time with".

Max Walker, Sporting Legend, Writer and Keynote Speaker

Most people spend most of their lives earning a living rather than
designing a life. At the Live your Passion seminar Keith Abraham
will help you take control of every aspect of your life, so that you
live a life filled will passion.

There are no impractical ideas that don't work in reality. No
hollow claims. No smoke and mirrors. Just real world strategies
that are proven to work famously well day-in-day-out by people
from all walks of life.

This is Keith Abraham as you have never seen him before. There
will be no holding back as he gives you the time proven techniques
of outstanding achievers and success strategies of the successful.
Keith's unwavering belief is you deserve the very best life has to
offer and it is now time that you stop selling yourself short and tap
into your true potential.

This one day seminar empowers you to achieve your untapped potential by giving you ...

- The 4 ways to have unwavering personal focus and a passion for excellence

- 6 steps to having Power, Passion and Pizzazz in your life

- The 23 vital factors for creating successful outcomes in your future and how to equip yourself so you believe you deserve it.

- The 4 parts of your personal success cycle and how to make it work every time for you.

- How to develop specific strategies for achieving your short term, medium term and long term goals.

- Understand the 5 ways to work smarter, make more $$$ and have loving supportive relationships.

- 10 ways to gain the unwavering self confidence so that you can achieve extraordinary things.

- How to create a plan to overcome ANY obstacle that stops you from achieving.

- How to remain focused on what counts in your personal and professional life.

- How to stop earning a living that keeps you on the poverty line and create a life filled with wealth and success.

- How to design the life you want with balance, achievement and success.

No-Risk, No Questions Asked, No Hidden Catches, "Love it or your Money Back" Guarantee

It's simple. Join us at the Live your Passion seminar and if at any time during or after the seminar you're not 100% delighted with the value of the material, or you're not happy for any other reason just let us know and we'll give you a full refund. No hidden catches. No questions asked.

What people say about Keith:

"I have never seen the team so enthusiastic about a presentation before!!!"
Rob Newbold, Sale & Marketing Manager, CSL Animal Health.

"I was stimulated, liberated, and ultimately more spirited."
Steven Jones, Team Leader Hobart Call Centre, Telstra

"Keith is an exceptional presenter who has a great ability to acquire the knowledge of the business and to deliver a dynamic and engaging presentation to the audience. Keith stands out as a professional who delivers long lasting business results every time and from my perspective the return on investment through enhanced skill and personal development has been significant."
Ian Andrew, General Manager, Personalised Plates Queensland

"Keith's contribution to our people's personal development has been phenomenal. He has been a catalyst for our people and organisation to achieve measurable gains in performance."
Jim Carlile - Human Resources Manager, Terry White Management Pty Ltd

"... Keith inspired and supported our audience beyond expectations. A passionate communicator and a pleasure to work with".

Belinda Vaughan - Assistant Marketing Manager, Agfa Gevaert Limited

"You have an amazing talent in explaining and presenting real theory with an energy which inspired and challenged our delegates to make real changes. The evidence of this value is in the feedback we continue to receive six weeks after the event, and the 'Keith-isms' which have filtered into some emails we've recently received."

Kathryn Snell - Communications and Public Relations Manager, Bakers Delight Holdings Ltd

See order form on opposite page to find out how to book.

Book now! One day Living Your Passion Seminar or email jill@keithabraham.com.au

☐ Yes, I'd like to invest in this life changing seminar ... Live Your Passion for $495.00 per person. I want to purchase _____ tickets @ $ _____
= Total $ _____

I am paying by:

☐ Cheque (please make cheques payable to People Pursuing a Passion P/L)

☐ Mastercard   ☐ Visa   ☐ American Express   ☐ Bankcard   ☐ Diners

Card no: ☐☐☐☐ ☐☐☐☐ ☐☐☐☐ ☐☐☐☐

Cardholder: _____ Expires: _____ / _____

AMEX ID: _____

Signature: _____

Company name: _____

Surname: _____ First name: _____

Address: _____ P/code: _____

Phone: _____ Fax: _____

Email: _____

Post to: People Pursuing a Passion, P.O. Box 865 Robina QLD. 4226

Website: www.keithabraham.com.au Email: seminar@keithabraham.com.au

Keith Abraham – Inspirational Information Pack

PACK 1. Total value $108.95

"Power Passion Pizzazz" by Keith Abraham
52 Inspirational Messages to keep you motivated in this handy desk or coffee table size book. How to have the Power to Pursue; the Passion to Fulfill and the Pizzazz to Live!
RRP $19.95

"Be Happy Book" by Rowena McEvoy
This book contains 105 simple ways to BE HAPPY. It shows you can smile, laugh, be successful and be the best person you can be everyday. WARNING, If you apply all 105 ways you will BE HAPPY!
RRP $20.00

"How to have Power Passion & Pizzazz, Online Monthly Ideas" by Keith Abraham
This program has been designed to give you a monthly reminder of why it is important to stay focused in your personal and professional life. The monthly inspirational ideas are designed to refocus you on the activities that count in your life.
RRP $69.00
PACK 1. Total Value $~~108.95~~ $40.00

PACK 2. Invest an extra $35.00

"How to have a Balanced Life CD" by Keith Abraham, Simon Tupman, Robyn Henderson.
How to make lifestyle choices, and design the life you want to live, lead and love! Gain insights into the choices you have TODAY to create a great lifestyle; Learn how to take the FIRST STEPS towards your lifestyle choices; Gain the CONFIDENCE to put a plan of action into place; Understand what is STOPPING YOU from capturing what life has to offer you TODAY; Hear how to become a more confident DECISION MAKER; Practical TIME PROVEN strategies, solutions and ideas on how to LIVE A LIFE worth living. **PLUS** Power, Passion, Pizzazz Book, Be Happy Book, Monthly Online Power, Passion & Pizzazz e-course to help you stay motivated.
RRP $49.95

"Lessons in Leadership" by Keith Abraham
This book is an Owners Manual for the rest of your life. Though the contributors are diverse, they are united by proven success and by a common theme. It gives you insights into business from ten of Australia's leading consultants. The unifying factor in the diversity of the chapters is that there is always room at the top.
RRP $27.50
PACK 2. Total Value $~~158.90~~ $75.00

PACK 3. Invest an extra $120.00

"Pursuing Your Passion Audio and Video CD" by Keith Abraham
Use these 1 hour video and audio on Creating loyal profitable customers to train your team. It reveals 47 tried and proven methods of increasing customer loyalty in your business as well as easy-to-use market-tested hints and tips that can be implemented in any business today which will dramatically increase your bottom-line profits. **PLUS** How to have a balanced life CD, Power, Passion, Pizzazz Book, Be Happy Book, Lessons in leadership & Monthly Online Power, passion & Pizzazz e-course to help you stay motivated.
RRP $129.00
PACK 3. Total Value $~~342.90~~ $195.00

Special Keith Abraham Offer. Take the lot for $~~342.90~~ $195.00

Keith Abraham – Business Building Pack

PACK 1. Total value $121.50

"Creating Loyal Profitable Customers" by Keith Abraham
Loyalty is something money can't buy! For many businesses, staying afloat is an everyday a struggle, but what they don't realise is that there are ways to work 'smarter' and make more profit without the backbreaking work.

RRP $25.00

"Masters of Networking" by Robyn Henderson
Building relationships for your pocketbook and soul - featuring Bill Gates, Deepak Chopra, Colin Powell, John Naisbitt and Robyn Henderson (to name a few of the authors). What is different about master networkers, how are their lives different? What actions lead them to greater success than the rest of us? All your networking questions answered.

RRP $27.50

"Creating Loyal Profitable Customers, Online Weekly Loyalty Ideas" by Keith Abraham
This program has been designed to give you a weekly reminder of many great Loyalty Ideas which come from Keith's book 'Creating Loyal Profitable Customers'. The weekly loyalty ideas are designed to refocus you on the activities that count in your business.

RRP $69.00

PACK 1. Total Value ~~$121.50~~ $40.00

PACK 2. Invest an extra $35.00

"How to Increase Your Website Traffic by 100% in 30 Days" by Paul Klerck
This informatative CD by Paul Klerck Search Engine Optimiser and Keith Abraham will share with you the 10 fact that your website designer fails to tell you. You will learn: Avoid costly unproductive pitfalls when creating your website, how to increase your website traffic, create customer loyalty online plus much much more. **PLUS** Customer loyalty book, Lessons in Leadership book, Online loyalty ideas.

RRP $49.95

PACK 2. Total Value ~~$171.45~~ $75.00

PACK 3. Invest an extra $100.00

"Customer Loyalty Audio & Video CD" by Keith Abraham
Use these 1 hour video and audio on Creating loyal profitable customers to train your team. It reveals 47 tried and proven methods of increasing customer loyalty in your business as well as easy-to-use market-tested hints and tips that can be implemented in any business today which will dramatically increase your bottom-line profits. **PLUS** Customer loyalty book, Lessons in Leadership book, Online loyalty ideas, How to increase your website traffic by 100% in 30 days by Paul Klerck.

RRP $129.00

PACK 3. Total Value ~~$300.45~~ $175.00

Keith Abraham – Business Building Pack cont...

PACK 4. Invest an extra $252
"Customer Loyalty Manual" by Keith Abraham
If you want to take your business to the next level of success, this program is a must. A 2 hour video, 2 x 60 min audio tape with a comprehensive Customer Loyalty manual. You will discover leading-edge business building strategies, whether you are a Sales Person, Manager, Executive, Home-Based Business Owner, Customer Service Person, Franchisee or Entreprenuer. **PLUS** Customer loyalty video & audio CD, Customer loyalty book, Lessons in Leadership book, Online loyalty ideas, How to increase your website traffic by 100% in 30 days by Paul Klerck.

RRP $295.00

PACK 4. Total Value ~~$595.45~~ **$427.00**

Special Keith Abraham Offer. Take the lot for ~~$595.45~~ $427.00

See order form on opposite page or visit our website
www.keithabraham.com.au

Order Form

☐ YES, I want to buy the Inspirational Information Pack.

Total Amount: $A _____

☐ YES, I want to buy the Business Information Pack.

Total Amount: $A _____

Name: _____ Date: / /

Company: _____

Postal Address: _____

Suburb: _____ State: _____ Postcode: _____

Email: _____

Method of Payment:

☐ Visa ☐ Mastercard ☐ Bankcard ☐ Diners ☐ Amex ☐ Cheque

Postage/handling $7.50 per pack, individual items $5.50 Credit card will say People Pursuing A Passion

Card Number: ☐☐☐☐ ☐☐☐☐ ☐☐☐☐ ☐☐☐☐

Expiry: /   Name on Card: _____

Signature: _____

Office use only:

☐ Received at event   Send to: ☐ Posted product

People Pursuing a Passion, PO Box 3152, Yeronga   QLD   4104

Website: www.keithabraham.com.au   Email: keith@keithabraham.com.au

Your notes

Your notes

Your notes

Your notes

_____

_____

_____

_____

_____

_____

_____

_____

_____

_____

_____

_____

_____

_____

_____

_____

_____

_____

_____

_____

_____

_____

_____